Building Healthy Communities
through Medical-Religious
Partnerships

BUILDING HEALTHY COMMUNITIES THROUGH MEDICAL-RELIGIOUS PARTNERSHIPS

W. Daniel Hale, Ph.D.
Professor, Department of Psychology
Stetson University
DeLand, Florida

and

Richard G. Bennett, M.D.
Associate Professor, Department of Medicine
The Johns Hopkins University School of Medicine
Baltimore, Maryland

The Johns Hopkins University Press
Baltimore & London

This book was brought to publication with the generous assistance of the
Catherine J. McGinnis Family Foundation.

The Johns Hopkins University Press
2715 North Charles Street
Baltimore, Maryland 21218-4363
www.press.jhu.edu

Library of Congress Cataloging-in-Publication Data will be found at the end of
this book.
A catalog record for this book is available from the British Library.

ISBN 0-8018-6347-3 (pbk.)

To our parents

William and Frances Hale

Wilford and Evelyn Bennett

Contents

Preface

This book was written for members of religious congregations and professionals involved in health care who want to see religious and medical communities work together to enhance congregational and community health. People who believe that hospitals, medical professionals, and religious congregations should join forces to minister to the health needs of the community will find in this book not only support for their belief but also detailed information and advice on programs that have been proven successful in a diverse group of congregations and communities.

This book provides the blueprint for building effective programs. It includes practical and easily accessible information for establishing health education programs as well as important topics to consider. There are examples of specific programs, including various congregational programs, as well as information on additional resources available from national organizations. The major disease-specific topics covered include coronary heart disease, hypertension, cancer, diabetes, depression, and dementia. These are among the most common chronic diseases for which educational programs are needed. Prevention programs on influenza and pneumonia, accidents and falls, and medication management are also described, as well as the topic of advance directives.

Additionally, we present a section on the concept of a patient advocacy or health partners program. This program helps train individuals within a congregation to assist other members with chronic illnesses who may not have relatives or close friends to help them navigate a complex health system. Although informal programs may be in place in some congregations, this section describes a systematic approach for establishing a health partners program and covers important topics that should be included in the training of patient advocates.

In the final section, we offer suggestions on how to identify congregational members who are likely to be effective health educators and advocates and who will find participation in these health ministries gratifying. We also have included a chapter by Barbara Pearson, a lay health educator who has established a vibrant health ministry program in her congregation. She offers her perspective on the challenges and rewards of such a program.

The text is based on work undertaken in central Florida during the last six years that has resulted in collaboration between local health care systems and religious organizations. Although the concept for these partnerships was envisioned by academicians and catalyzed by foundation support and the ongoing involvement of a university-based educator, the strategies outlined provide the direction for any health care organization or religious congregation to move forward with a program in its own community. Congregations that already have a health ministry, perhaps under the direction of a parish nurse, can expand their offerings and reach more members by training interested volunteers to become effective lay health educators and advocates.

In our experience, we have found that hospitals of all sizes and religious congregations of all faiths can indeed work together to advance community health. The programs described in this book began when we and a small group of hospital administrators and physicians committed to building a healthier community invited clergy to join us in developing innovative community health programs that would be based in congregations. We did not know what to expect when we issued this invitation. We did not know if we would succeed, but we did believe that the effort was worthwhile. We knew that this was the only way to answer our questions: Would clergy be willing and able to find energetic volunteers in their congregations who could be trained as lay health educators and patient advocates? Would doctors, nurses, pharmacists, and other health professionals volunteer their time to train the congregational volunteers and then later to serve as guest speakers and consultants for local congregations? Would members of local congregations and people in neighborhoods surrounding these congregations participate in the health programs?

The answer to each of these questions was a resounding Yes! Clergy found outstanding volunteers who were eager to learn strategies for addressing the health needs of their congregations and communities. Doctors and other health professionals offered to provide instruction and advice to volunteers. Later these professionals and many of their colleagues went out into the congregations to offer information and services. Programs on heart disease, cancer, diabetes, depression, dementia, and many other important topics were offered. And the people came to listen and receive assistance.

Word of these programs spread. More congregations wanted to participate. Soon volunteers from a diverse group of religious institutions had been trained, and community-based health programs were being offered in Christian and Jewish congregations. The programs were especially successful in reaching into African-American and Hispanic communities. We discovered that we were able to overcome many of the barriers that are frequently encountered when medical institutions and professionals try to reach members of minority communities. By listening carefully to the concerns of clergy and lay leaders in these congregations, and by consistently demonstrating our commitment to empower members of their community, we were able to forge strong alliances. Not only were we invited into communities that have been hard to reach but also our efforts were multiplied greatly by the work of committed, energetic volunteers who shared our vision of enhancing the health of these communities.

Hospitals in other communities heard about this work. They asked for similar programs in their communities. Clergy in these communities were contacted, congregational volunteers were selected, and medical professionals offered their time to provide training for the volunteers and later became active in congregational programs. Through the efforts of these medical professionals and dedicated volunteers, people in various congregations and communities were given the tools they needed to take charge of their health.

It was exciting and gratifying to witness these developments. Baptists, Catholics, Presbyterians, Lutherans, Methodists, Jews, Episcopalians, and Muslims were working together with the common goal of ministering to the health needs of their congregations and communities. They were being assisted by physicians, nurses, pharmacists, dietitians, psychologists, physical therapists, and other health professionals who shared the same goal. Through their efforts, valuable medical information and resources were being brought to their communities.

Examples of these programs, along with numerous suggestions for strategies and resources that can be used in congregational health ministries, can be found throughout the book. We hope that many who read this book will be inspired to take on the richly rewarding task of developing medical-religious partnerships in their communities. The programs described can serve as a good starting point for joint efforts between hospitals and religious congregations, but they should serve only as a beginning. Once members of religious congregations and representatives of health care organizations come together with the common mission of serving and empowering members of their community, they will discover innumerable opportunities. The needs of every community are great, but so are the resources that are created when religious and medical communities unite.

A PERSONAL NOTE

Premature illness, disability, and death. These words may sound theoretical or academic to many people, but to me (WDH) they have a very personal and powerful meaning. I cannot think about the concept of premature illness without thinking of my late father, a physically imposing (six feet four inches tall) and dynamic man. For most of my childhood and adolescence, he appeared to be in good health and to have almost limitless energy. Although he worked long hours as an executive at a rapidly expanding business, he always found time to devote to his family and his church. I felt that he was an outstanding role model, and I planned to pattern much of my life after his.

In 1966, when I was still a teenager, I discovered that the appearance of good health can be deceiving. During that year, my father, who was not yet 44 years old, suffered a major heart attack. The man who previously had seemed almost invincible was now seriously wounded. He was fortunate to receive good medical care at an excellent hospital and was able to return to work and many of his previous activities. Following the recommendations of his physician, he made significant changes in his lifestyle and seemed to be enjoying life again. He began exercising more, watched his diet, lost weight, and found ways to manage better the stress in his life. However, a little more than a decade later, he encountered a major crisis at work and gradually gave up many of the healthy practices he had been following. In 1980, at the age of 57, he had another heart attack. This one was more severe and damaging. In fact, the damage was so great that he was unable to return to work. At an age when many men are at the height of their productivity, my father was permanently disabled.

My father's disability affected much more than his capacity to work. He and my mother could no longer travel as extensively as they liked. There were no more cross-country trips and visits to the national parks they loved. Nor could he play much with my two daughters. His congestive heart failure made it impossible for him to take them on long walks around the neighborhood or accompany them to playgrounds and nearby theme parks.

In 1982 my son was born. My wife and I decided to name him after my father, who was thrilled to have a grandson living near him. My father was eager to watch him grow and listen to reports of each new developmental milestone he reached. But he had less than two years to spend with his grandson. In 1984, while resting at home, my father died of heart failure. The man I loved and admired so much died before he reached his 62nd birthday. I was not yet 34 and my son was three months shy of his second birthday. My son, who is like his grandfather in so many ways, has no memory of him. Like his grandfather, he loves baseball. (Unlike his father, he is very good at it.) Now 17, he has been playing baseball for more than a decade, and every time he gets a hit or makes an outstanding defensive play, I think about how much my father would have enjoyed watching him. I always feel a certain sadness, knowing that these two people never had the opportunity to develop a relationship that would have been so gratifying to each.

A heart attack at 43, a crippling heart attack at 57, heart failure at 61 — these are the events I recall when I think of premature illness, disability, and death. They are not abstract terms; they are very real and very personal. They represent painful losses for me and my children. I believe that my family's church could have made a critical difference in my father's health. A comprehensive health insurance policy and good medical treatment provided by a caring physician and a respected hospital were not enough. My father needed a steady flow of reliable information about heart disease and ongoing support from the people he respected and trusted. He and the people to whom he looked for advice and encouragement needed a better understanding of heart disease and what they could do to slow its progression. Perhaps more than anything, my father needed to be regularly reminded of the importance of following health-enhancing practices and avoiding activities and situations that were potentially harmful to his health. I am convinced that a church-sponsored health ministry could have provided these resources and given my father at least a few more years to enjoy life and to enrich the lives of others.

Acknowledgments

We could not have written a book about community partnerships and programs without the assistance and goodwill of many people. The programs we developed were truly collaborative endeavors, and we want to thank all of the health professionals, clergy, and members of religious congregations who gave of their time, energy, and talents.

We are particularly grateful to John Burton, M.D., Mason F. Lord Professor of Medicine and Director of the Division of Geriatric Medicine and Gerontology at the Johns Hopkins University School of Medicine, for his many valuable contributions. Dr. Burton encouraged us to undertake this project and generously offered us his wisdom and support throughout the years we have worked on it.

We are deeply indebted to Mr. and Mrs. William E. O'Neill, of Daytona Beach, for their steadfast interest and support. The programs we initially designed could easily have gone no farther than the idea stage if it had not been for their generosity and efforts on our behalf.

Halifax Medical Center in Daytona Beach gave us our first opportunity to test our ideas in the "real world." Ron Rees, Herb Kerman, M.D., Dan Lang, and John E. Evans were especially helpful in making the arrangements for our first training programs. Neil Oslos, M.D., a member of the faculty at the Halifax Medical Center Family Practice Residency Program, served as the principal medical advisor for these training programs and, along with Don Stoner, M.D., and Greg Favis, M.D., assisted in developing the curriculum for the first lay health educator training program.

An opportunity to expand our work into other communities and explore ways to further develop medical-religious partnerships arose when Joan

Salmons and Tom Werner, of Florida Hospital in Orlando, invited us to bring our programs to their health care system. They enthusiastically embraced the concept of training volunteers from local congregations as lay health educators and advocates and brought together a talented group of professionals to coordinate the training programs. Laura Orem, Shelly Siebenlist, and Pamela Jansen were key members of this group, and we are indebted to them for their contributions. It was through one of the programs sponsored by Florida Hospital that we met Barbara Pearson, Charles Horton, D.Min., and Tom Allerton, Ed.D., of College Park Baptist Church. These individuals, working together as a team, built a strong health ministry program that has served as a model for other congregations and gave us a better understanding of what committed clergy and lay leaders can accomplish.

We also want to acknowledge the assistance of many people at Stetson University. Dwaine Cochran, Ph.D., Dick Kindred, Ph.D., and other members of the Department of Psychology have provided direct and indirect support for our work. Clyde Fant, Th.D., Professor of Religious Studies, and Paul Langston, S.M.D., Professor of Church Music, Emeritus, were among the first to see the potential of congregational health ministries and encourage us to develop these programs. Special thanks are due Denise Heist of the Center for the Study of Aging and Health for her many and varied contributions. She assisted in the preparation of program materials, maintained regular contact with volunteers from local congregations and representatives of community agencies, made arrangements for special events, and found creative solutions to seemingly insurmountable problems. Kim Norman, who served for many years in the Human Resources Department as a highly effective health advocate for members of the Stetson community, contributed in many ways to our project. In addition to offering valuable advice about the health needs and resources in the community, she assisted in the preparation of materials and organizing of special events. In another role, that as wife of one of the authors (WDH), she sacrificed many nights and weekends as work on the manuscript consumed more and more time.

We are also grateful to Bill Allen, M.Div., J.D., of the Program in Medical Ethics, Law, and Humanities at the University of Florida College of Medicine, and Dianne Dixon, both of whom offered helpful suggestions for programs and the manuscript. Finally, we wish to thank our editor, Wendy Harris, for her encouragement and guidance.

Building Healthy Communities
through Medical-Religious
Partnerships

Introduction

The health care system in the United States continues to undergo dramatic evolution. Although currently much attention is being paid to the perceived abuses and shortcomings of managed care organizations, these same organizations and many health care providers who are entering the managed care business are expanding their focus to include disease prevention as well as the treatment of illness. These care-management strategies recognize that the historic approach of treating an acute illness in the hospital and providing uncoordinated longitudinal care following hospital discharge was not ideal. There is a need to develop new approaches to improve disease management, prevent illness, and educate patients and their families, and this need will increase as the number of older adults with multiple chronic diseases continues to grow in the coming years. Care-management strategies focused on patient education and prevention will be the foundation of U.S. health care in the future.

Although health care organizations have grown larger through mergers in many regions of the United States in recent years, the formation of these partnerships alone has not usually resulted in dramatic changes in the delivery of health care services. Even organizations focused on improving the management of chronic diseases have relied on forging partnerships between and among hospitals, physician groups, nursing homes, and home care providers, and they have paid less attention to coordinating care among the providers or educating large groups of patients and their families. This book describes a new approach to partnerships: the formation of alliances between religious congregations and health care organizations.

These alliances are designed to carry out community-based education and advocacy programs targeted at disease management and prevention.

The need for such programs is great and will be recognized by any religious organization that carefully considers the needs of its members. In every church, synagogue, or mosque, there are individuals with unmet health care needs. These members and their families have health care problems that education and advocacy programs can address. Programs focused on the management of specific diseases such as high blood pressure and diabetes increase everyone's understanding of these problems and can alert people to the need for identifying these conditions as early as possible to minimize future complications. And since the management of one family member's health problem often involves the help and encouragement of everyone in the family, religious organizations can play an important role in facilitating familial support systems.

As health care organizations look beyond their own walls, they too will see the need to develop more education and patient support systems in the community. Partnering with local religious congregations can provide a new stage for educating potential patients. These partnerships can augment typical hospital outreach programs such as lecture series in a hospital auditorium or at a local senior center. In addition, partnering with respected leaders from a nearby congregation often guarantees a larger audience than would be assembled through advertisement. Finally, these religious leaders, through both surveys of and conversations with the members of their congregations, can help the health care organization tailor programs to meet actual needs.

This book provides the tools to establish these partnerships and create successful programs. In each community, a leader will need to act as the champion for ensuring the success of the partnership. In some locales, it may be a hospital administrator or physician who can see the benefit of such programs and will advocate the forging of partnerships that will result in outreach from the health care organization. In other communities, interested clergy or congregational lay leaders may assume this role and work to build a partnership with a local hospital. In addition, this book explains why religious organizations should be interested in such partnerships if approached by a health care organization, as well as why the health care organization should be interested if approached by clergy or religious leaders.

Our premise is that partnerships between medical and religious organizations can materially contribute to shaping healthier communities. Such partnerships can harness the energies of committed members of religious communities and couple that energy with information and resources provided by health care professionals. The success of such programs will be measured not only by the numbers of lectures and programs carried out within individual churches, synagogues, and mosques but also by the actual improvement in health care outcomes for the members and their families.

This idea of establishing alliances between religious and medical institutions developed during a period in which there was a significant growth in interest in the relationship between various dimensions of religion or spirituality and health. This heightened interest has taken many forms. Medical researchers have studied the relationship between religious commitment and both physical and mental health, with numerous published reports indicating that religious faith has a beneficial effect. Many medical schools now offer courses in which the role of religion in health and health care is explored. Conferences on spirituality and health draw hundreds of medical professionals and religious leaders from throughout the United States. Books exploring religious commitment and health can be found in almost every major bookstore and attract both professional and lay audiences. (See "Suggested Readings" on this topic.) Although this book does not discuss this phenomenon specifically, the development of health programs within religious communities described herein seems to be a part of this larger movement toward finding links between religion and health, and will no doubt be energized by the current renewed interest.

This growing interest in the relationship between religion and health has come at a critical time. We are at a point where many health care leaders, recognizing the complex and immense health-related challenges our society now faces, are eager to explore cooperative efforts between medical and religious institutions. They realize that medical institutions must develop new strategies and resources if they are to be successful in meeting the health needs of the twenty-first century. Major medical centers and community hospitals cannot meet these needs by themselves. They will need to do more than treat the seriously ill. They will need to take the lead in building and maintaining healthy communities. To accomplish this task, they must find ways to reach out into their communities and connect with people. They need to reach out to healthy people and provide them with the information and resources they need to maintain their health. Hospitals must also reach out to people who have chronic illnesses and give them the information and support they need to manage their illnesses and maintain their independence.

To reach and maintain contact with people, hospitals need partners. They need to work closely with institutions that are deeply rooted in the community and that are trusted by the people in the community. Hospitals need to develop alliances with institutions that have a strong tradition of caring for others and that attract people who identify with this tradition.

Churches, synagogues, mosques, and temples clearly fit this description. They have the community resources and networks that hospitals need. Just as important, they have the altruistic traditions and values that are at the heart of community-based health programs. No community institutions are better suited to serve as partners for hospitals. This is especially true for addressing the health needs of older adults and families who have the responsibility of caring for older adults. Whereas most children and adolescents can be reached through school-based health promotion programs and most young and middle-aged adults can be reached through work-site initiatives, there are few places other than religious institutions where large numbers of older adults regularly gather. In fact, two-thirds of adults aged 50 and over—the age group likely to be affected by chronic illnesses—are members of religious institutions and attend religious services monthly or even more frequently.

The programs and materials presented in this book are by no means exhaustive. Many other programs can be sponsored by religious congregations, and religious and medical institutions can work together in many other ways to enhance community health. The most important point to remember is that there has never been a better time to explore innovative and collaborative efforts to minister to the health needs of communities. We are in the midst of a fundamental change in the way people are conceptualizing and organizing health care. Health care leaders are awakening to the fact that they need to reach out into the community through trusted institutions, and religious leaders are learning that they can ask for assistance and support from medical institutions. We encourage you to take the initiative to bring religious and medical communities even closer together.

THE RELIGIOUS CONGREGATION
AND HEALTH CARE

1

The Religious Congregation
and Preventive Medicine

Sunday morning. The worship service at the rural Catholic Hispanic mission is over, and more than a hundred parishioners who attended the service are now lined up to be vaccinated against influenza. Nurses from the health department and volunteers from a large Catholic church are ready to give an influenza shot free of charge to anyone who requests it.

Monday morning. An 81-year-old woman who has multiple health problems is receiving assistance from a retired schoolteacher. Both are members of a Lutheran church. The retired teacher has been trained by doctors, pharmacists, nurses, and a psychologist to serve as a patient advocate. Using materials she received in the hospital-sponsored training program, the patient advocate works with the patient to compile a list of concerns to discuss with her doctor. Then she accompanies the patient to the appointment, helps her explain these concerns to the doctor, records the doctor's comments and recommendations, and assists the patient in organizing her medications at home. She also makes arrangements to contact the patient on a regular basis to be certain that she is taking her medications as prescribed.

Tuesday afternoon. Fifty people, drawn from Lutheran, Presbyterian, Christian and Missionary Alliance, and Episcopal congregations, as well as from the community at large, have gathered in the sanctuary of the Episcopal church. They are there to learn more about how they can maintain control over important medical decisions by using living wills and other types of advance directives. A physician and an attorney provide the group with valuable general information and then talk with individual members of the audience who need more specific information.

Wednesday evening. The members of a men's organization at a Baptist church in an African-American community are attending their regular midweek meeting. Tonight they have a special speaker, an African-American physician who warns them of the dangers of prostate cancer and offers advice on detecting and treating this type of cancer. He also provides them with information on cancer services in the community.

Thursday afternoon. More than a hundred people have gathered in the fellowship hall of the Presbyterian church to hear a physician speak on hypertension and heart disease. He is joined by volunteer nurses, who are conducting blood pressure checks, and representatives of the American Heart Association, who are distributing information on ways to prevent, detect, and treat these conditions. After his presentation, the physician meets individually with those who request additional information.

Friday evening. A psychiatrist is speaking to members of the temple who are attending the Shabbat service. His goal is to alert people of the dangers of undetected and untreated depression. After describing the symptoms of depression, he offers them hope and guidance by explaining how depression can be treated effectively by psychotherapy, medication, or a combination of the two. The psychiatrist stays for the reception after the service and speaks individually with people seeking more information or advice.

Saturday morning. More than fifty people have gathered at the Catholic church to learn more about dementia and depression. A neurologist speaks first, describing dementia and explaining the treatments and services that are available in the community. A psychologist then provides information on how to recognize depression and the treatments for it. After the presentations, both speakers meet individually with people who need additional information.

Although it is not surprising that religious congregations would offer programs that minister to the physical and emotional needs of their members and the community at large, it may seem surprising that medical institutions and professionals would be interested in working hand-in-hand with the congregations. Why is this happening? Why are doctors and nurses getting out of the hospital and into the community? How do such programs fit in with the current mission of hospitals and the changing health care scene?

What we are witnessing is a growing recognition that we cannot afford to have a health care system that responds only when people are sick and disabled. The economic and human costs of waiting for people to become seriously ill or disabled before they are provided with medical services are too great. We must find better ways to apply the medical knowledge we have acquired. To achieve this, we need to adopt the principles and methods of *preventive medicine*. This field is dedicated to preventing, or at least greatly reducing the risk of, premature illness, disability, and death. The key to effective preventive medicine programs is getting medical information and resources to people in a timely and easy-to-use fashion. The goal is to have everyone acquire a better understanding of what can be done to maintain health and ensure functional independence. This is where religious congregations fit in so well.

This chapter introduces the basic concepts of preventive medicine and illustrates how these can be incorporated into the life and mission of religious congregations.

PREVENTIVE MEDICINE PROGRAMS

Preventive practices and interventions are generally organized into three categories or levels: primary, secondary, and tertiary. The following sections provide descriptions and examples of programs at each of these levels.

Primary Prevention

The goal of primary prevention is to prevent the development of disease. By engaging in health-enhancing practices and avoiding health-compromising activities, people can greatly reduce their risk of developing various chronic diseases and conditions. Included in this category are both lifestyle modifications and immunizations. Some examples are as follows:

- Giving up smoking
- Exercising regularly

- Eating properly
- Preventing injuries
- Obtaining vaccinations against influenza, pneumonia, and tetanus

One of the greatest challenges facing any organization sponsoring a primary prevention informational program is that many people do not pay attention to health matters until a serious illness or injury strikes. It is not easy to persuade people who are feeling healthy that they need to make lifestyle changes (e.g., diet, exercise, and cessation of smoking), especially when there are no immediate apparent benefits. Even when individuals believe that ignoring such advice may have negative consequences on their health, the changes they need to make may seem too great or too costly because these consequences may not occur until much later in their lives and therefore do not significantly impact their current lifestyle.

Religious institutions have certain advantages when sponsoring primary prevention programs. First, they can incorporate information about primary prevention practices into regularly scheduled programs. In this way, they have an already "built-in" audience. Second, they can present the information in different formats and at various times. This is important since one message alone is seldom sufficient to produce lasting changes in long-standing behavioral patterns. Most people need to hear such messages several times. Third, most religious congregations have members of all ages. This allows them to schedule intergenerational programs on health matters. They can encourage older adults, especially those who have chronic illnesses, to bring their children and even grandchildren to an informational program. Children and young adults are more likely to listen to and heed advice on illness prevention measures when they can see first-hand the impact of chronic diseases.

Example of a Congregational Primary Prevention Program

A program that encourages older adults to get annual influenza vaccinations is a simple and yet highly effective primary prevention program you can sponsor for your congregation and community. In a typical year, there are approximately 10,000 to 20,000 deaths and 150,000 hospitalizations resulting from influenza and its complications. In spite of the grave dangers associated with influenza and substantial evidence for the effectiveness of the vaccine, large numbers of older adults fail to get annual vaccinations. Educational programs sponsored jointly by congregations and respected health organizations can increase the number of vaccinations for and decrease the number of hospitalizations and deaths due to influenza. (For more information on this topic, see chapter 12.)

Secondary Prevention

The goal of secondary prevention is early detection of disease. By identifying a disease through medical screenings before its symptoms become evident and providing treatment for the disease before it can advance further, the impact can be reduced. Once a disease or condition has been detected, interventions may include strictly medical measures or some of the lifestyle modifications listed in the section on primary prevention. Recommended screenings generally include the following:

- Breast cancer
- Colorectal cancer
- Skin cancer
- Hypertension
- Hypercholesterolemia
- Depression and potential for suicide

Time and transportation can be barriers to secondary prevention. Many people complain that they do not have the time in their busy schedules to participate in medical screenings and counseling, particularly when they are feeling healthy. Other individuals, especially many older adults, may have the time for screenings but find it difficult to arrange transportation. Religious congregations can help people overcome both of these barriers by arranging for screenings to be conducted on-site and in conjunction with regularly scheduled congregational activities. Hospitals and home health agencies can be enlisted to assist in these screenings. If you cannot arrange to have screenings conducted in your congregational facilities, you can still facilitate the screenings by arranging for transportation to and from the local hospital or medical laboratory.

Example of a Congregational Secondary Prevention Program

A simple, inexpensive secondary prevention program that can be sponsored by a religious congregation is one in which volunteer nurses provide blood pressure checks after the worship service. Little time and equipment are needed for this program, but it can yield meaningful results. By identifying people with high blood pressure and encouraging them to take appropriate measures to bring their blood pressure under control, you can reduce the incidence of heart attacks and strokes. Announcements in congregational bulletins and from respected congregational leaders can increase the number of people participating in and benefiting from this program. (For more information on this type of program, see chapter 5.)

Tertiary Prevention

The goal of tertiary prevention is to reduce complications and disabilities associated with existing disease. Patients and their families need to learn how to manage illnesses effectively. Appropriate management can help patients live longer and maintain their independence and quality of life. These are some preventive measures at the tertiary level:

- Identifying and using appropriate medical services
- Complying with recommendations about medication
- Using community resources to enhance functional health
- Sponsoring support groups for patients and families

Religious congregations are ideal for numerous types of tertiary prevention programs. Many people who have a chronic condition fail to receive appropriate treatments and related services because they do not know about various community resources. Clergy and lay leaders are usually aware of community medical services and other community agencies, often serving in leadership roles in these organizations. They can compile and pass along the information to members who need these services. Also, in order to ensure that members who live alone are doing well, many congregations have programs in which volunteers regularly check up on them by telephone. These volunteers can also be easily trained to use these contacts to remind members about their medication. Support groups for patients or families also fit well within the mission and ministry of most congregations.

Example of a Congregational Tertiary Prevention Program

One way a congregation can assist in tertiary prevention is to sponsor a support group for people with a specific disease or for their families experiencing illness-related stress. These groups can be helpful in many ways. Some people find it difficult to follow through with their treatment regimens on a consistent basis once the crisis seems to have passed. For example, some heart patients will revert to unhealthy dietary practices or abandon regular exercise programs once they feel they have recovered from a heart attack. Support groups can give these people and their families and caregivers the assistance and support they need to maintain their new regimens. Support groups can also help patients and their loved ones cope with some of the limitations and emotional aspects of an illness. Often new coping strategies can be learned from other members of the group.

2

Congregational
Health Education Programs

One of the most valuable and meaningful ministries that can be offered to a congregation and community is a proactive health education program. Information is at the heart of both health promotion and illness management. People of all ages, even children, need to know more about health, illnesses, and medical care. Most of the life-limiting and life-threatening diseases encountered in middle or late adulthood have their roots in earlier years. Members of your congregation and community need clear, reliable information about the steps they can take to reduce their risks of developing illnesses, and individuals who already have medical conditions need reliable information about how they can effectively treat or manage their conditions.

LINKING PEOPLE AND INFORMATION

Physicians, psychologists, and other researchers in the field of preventive medicine have developed a large body of scientific information about the steps people can take to prevent illnesses or reduce their impact. There is reliable information about the activities or practices that increase the odds of staying healthy as well as the ones that increase the odds of developing chronic illnesses or conditions. There are also well-established methods for detecting many diseases in their early stages, thus limiting their harmful effects.

Most of this information about health promotion, early detection programs, and illness management is uncomplicated and easy for people to comprehend. You do not have to be very knowledgeable about the biological or medical aspects of most illnesses to understand what types of activities will enhance your health and what types may compromise your health. Nor do you have to understand exactly how medical examinations are analyzed to receive the benefits of regular monitoring of certain key measures of your health.

Although most of the information we need about health matters is easy to understand, too many of us fail to take advantage of it. Either we do not obtain the necessary information or we fail to act on it. Why? The reasons are different for different people, and we need to understand and be sensitive to these reasons before we plan and implement a health education program.

BARRIERS TO ILLNESS PREVENTION

It is important to recognize that some people simply are not motivated to seek out information on health matters until a medical crisis arises. As long as they feel well, they are not interested in reading materials or attending programs on health issues. These individuals either are not aware of or do not care about the eventual consequences of their health-compromising actions.

Some individuals say they ignore information on health matters because they are confused by the various warnings and recommendations, which often seem contradictory to them—they do not know what to believe.

For others, they believe the information they have heard is reliable, but they cannot get motivated to act on it. They know that modifying some aspects of their lifestyle would be beneficial, but they cannot make the necessary changes. Sometimes they are simply too busy with other responsibilities.

Other people know what course of action they should take and make a decision to follow up on it, but then have difficulty staying on track. This is not surprising since most individuals find it hard to make lasting changes unless they receive regular reminders and ongoing encouragement and support.

OVERCOMING BARRIERS TO ILLNESS PREVENTION

Whatever the reasons, it is clear that too many people fail to use valuable information on health to their advantage. In fact, one of the greatest challenges in health care is finding an effective means of delivering important health information directly to the people who need it most, persuading them that they will benefit from this information, and providing the ongoing support they need to adhere to well-established prevention and treatment regimens. We must find innovative and appealing ways of reaching people with the information they need to maintain their health and independence.

Our work with many congregations has convinced us that religious institutions, through their professional and lay leaders, can play a critical role in bringing information and people together. Congregational leaders can reach people before they encounter a medical crisis. Furthermore, they can present the information in a manner that can be understood and appreciated by the members of their congregations and communities, and they can design informational programs that overcome many of the obstacles encountered in most community health education programs. These leaders have the potential to empower people by giving them the knowledge and tools they need to maintain their health and independence.

Although congregational leaders have many tangible and intangible resources they can utilize in their efforts to minister to the health needs of their congregations, they still face some significant challenges. Effective health education programs require a multifaceted, proactive approach. You have to do more than simply place attractive brochures in the pews.

First, you have to get the attention of the people. This is not always an easy task, but somehow you must reach out to them and convince them that you have information they need to hear. Second, you need to persuade them that there are actions they can take from which they will receive personal health benefits. Third, you must convince them that the benefits of their actions will outweigh the costs and burdens. Fourth, you need to bring them together in support of each other as they work to adopt and maintain their health-enhancing actions.

THE HEALTH BELIEF MODEL

Perhaps the most useful model to use in your planning is the health belief model (for more information, see the suggested readings). This simple model, consisting of four basic components, can help you organize the presentation of information such that it will have the greatest impact on your audiences. These four components are presented next, followed by an example that applies the health belief model to hypertension.

First, you must convince people that they are susceptible to a disease or condition. People who are not aware that they are vulnerable to a particular disease are not likely to take the correct steps to prevent its onset or detect it in the earliest stages.

Second, you need to persuade people that the disease or condition can have severe consequences. It is not enough for people to believe that they are susceptible to an illness; they must also realize that it can have severe consequences. They must see that a particular disease or condition could seriously limit their abilities and even shorten their life. People who believe that they may be susceptible to a particular illness but do not believe that the illness can have severe consequences are unlikely to make any modifications in their lifestyle or health practices.

Third, people must believe in the efficacy or power of the prevention or treatment regimens about which they will be learning. You need to convince people that there are steps they can take to reduce the risk of becoming ill or minimize the impact of a disease. If people believe that there are no effective treatments for a disease, they will see no reason to participate in early detection programs.

Fourth, people must believe that the benefits of illness prevention and treatment regimens outweigh the costs or burdens of those regimens. This point is often overlooked by health workers, who may not be aware of the perceived costs or burdens associated with certain actions. Although the benefits may seem obvious to health care professionals, many people feel that the costs associated with various treatments outweigh the benefits. Even small costs may be the primary reason that elderly or low-income persons do not seek services.

Health education programs that are designed with these objectives in mind are most likely to have an impact on members of your congregation and community.

THE HEALTH BELIEF MODEL AND HYPERTENSION

Hypertension, or high blood pressure, can illustrate how the health belief model can help you organize educational programs. First, you must realize that many people are unaware of the problem of high blood pressure or do not know they are susceptible to it. Some people believe that they are in good health as long as they do not have any painful symptoms. They do not think they need to concern themselves with getting their blood pressure checked unless they begin to feel ill. Therefore, the first step in educating and helping them to change their health practices is to find some way to convince them that they are susceptible to hypertension, even if they are not feeling ill or are not experiencing high levels of stress.

One way to help people understand that they are susceptible to hypertension is to give them information about its widespread prevalence. Once they realize that millions of people have hypertension but are unaware of their condition, they may be more willing to acknowledge the possibility that they too could have high blood pressure. This type of information may also help catch the attention of specific groups of people who are known to have high rates of hypertension, such as African Americans. Another way to reach and influence people is to give them examples of people similar to them who have high blood pressure. Often a few such personal examples are more effective than statistics.

Second, you need to persuade people that there are potentially severe consequences associated with hypertension. Individuals who are aware of the problem of hypertension but believe that there are no serious effects associated with it are not likely to monitor their blood pressure regularly and seek treatment should it be too high. They may view it as a condition that has little significance for their overall health. Other people may attempt to dismiss the risks associated with hypertension by saying, "I have to die of something." Often this is their way of avoiding a threatening subject, but such a statement also indicates that they are overlooking serious consequences other than death. These people need to be reminded that high blood pressure increases their risk of heart attack and stroke, both of which may leave them seriously disabled. Although they may survive, they may be left in a condition in which they are unable to participate in many of the activities they enjoy and find rewarding. The prospect of a long-term disability is often viewed as a more undesirable consequence than death.

Third, once you have made people understand that they are susceptible to hypertension and that it can have severe consequences, you need to persuade them that there are things they can do to help themselves. You need to offer hope and educate people about the steps to take to reduce the risk of hypertension and its potentially harmful consequences. They need to hear from reliable, authoritative sources that by making certain lifestyle modifications or taking medication, they can bring their blood pressure under control.

Fourth, you must be sensitive to people's perceptions about the cost of following the recommended prevention, monitoring, and treatment regimens for hypertension. Some people may believe the financial costs of treatment outweigh the benefits, especially if they are on a limited budget and have other important financial obligations. Others may fear that the side effects of the medication for their blood pressure will actually produce a poorer quality of life. Sometimes fears about the costs or negative effects of treatment are based on erroneous beliefs that can be corrected by providing accurate information from an authoritative source. However, in some situations, costs can be a real factor. In such cases, you may be able to give information about professionals or agencies that can provide less costly treatments or offer financial assistance.

MOTIVATING PEOPLE TO MAKE CHANGES

The health belief model can be quite useful in helping you to design programs and materials for members of your congregation. It should help you as you select topics and decide what type of information needs to be presented to your congregation or community. However, although many members of your congregation will appreciate your work, your efforts may not be warmly received or appreciated by all. You may encounter resistance or criticism from others in the congregation. Some individuals may feel that you are being critical or judgmental about them when you encourage them to make changes in their lifestyle. Often the people who have the greatest need to adopt new practices are the ones who are the most difficult to reach. It takes a sensitive and diplomatic approach in the presentation of information to overcome this resistance. Therefore, it is a good idea to know some basic principles and strategies that can be applied to situations in which you are encouraging people to adopt new health practices and to abandon, or at least alter, some long-standing habits.

William R. Miller and Stephen Rollnick provide in their book *Motivational Interviewing* a good model appropriate for work in congregations (see the suggested readings for additional information on this book). Although the principles and strategies they offer are generally used by counselors working on a one-to-one basis, they are also appropriate for working with groups of people who need encouragement as they seek to incorporate health-enhancing practices into their lifestyle and discard or reduce health-compromising habits.

The first principle of motivational interviewing is to *express empathy*. People are more open to change when they sense that you have a good understanding of their situation and the stresses and challenges they face in their life. They are more likely to listen to you and accept the information you are offering if they can tell that you understand how they feel. The steps you or your speakers recommend may seem both obvious and simple to you but may strike some people as overwhelming, at least given their current circumstances. To be truly empathic, it is necessary to listen carefully and with an open mind when these individuals express their feelings and concerns about what is being recommended. You need to be willing to put yourself in their position and be able to view life from their perspective. This does not mean you must agree with everything they say, but it does mean that you need to convey to them that you accept their actions, thoughts, and feelings without judging or criticizing them.

The second principle is to *develop discrepancy*. Although listening carefully and empathizing with people is an important and usually necessary first step in helping them to change, it is often not sufficient. For people to become motivated to actually make changes, they need to recognize that there is a discrepancy between where they are now with respect to health-enhancing practices and where they could be. They need to understand that they will fail to achieve some worthwhile goals if they continue their current practices. The awareness of this discrepancy is what can provide the fuel or energy for change. But it is important that this perceived discrepancy be between their current state and their goals, not yours. Therefore, you can be helpful by aiding them in identifying some goals that they truly value. These goals can vary tremendously. For some individuals, the goal of being able to live longer than their parents or with fewer health-related limitations may be best, whereas for others the goal of being able to maintain their health long enough to enjoy activities with their grandchildren may be the most important.

The third principle is to *avoid argumentation*. When people feel they are being directly attacked or criticized for "bad habits" or "problem behaviors," they are likely to become defensive and develop arguments that they believe justify their current practices. Even arguing that someone *should* have a particular goal or *should* follow certain practices can lead to resistance. Instead, keep the emphasis on the positive—the benefits of adopting some of the recommendations about how to become healthier. The objective of a good health education program is not to make people feel bad about their current health status but to inspire people to become healthier. You want to help people find their own reasons and rewards for avoiding health-compromising practices and adopting health-enhancing practices.

The fourth principle is to *roll with resistance*. Do not be surprised when people seem to ignore the information and services you are offering them. Not everyone is going to appreciate what you are trying to accomplish. But do not give up. Be flexible. Approach the topic from a different perspective, or focus on another topic. If people object to your approach or seem uninterested, ask them what type of information they want or what format for health education programs is the most appealing. Listen to their feedback and involve them in your planning process. In most situations, your audience can give you helpful advice about how to approach them.

The fifth principle is to *support self-efficacy*. People need to develop the belief that they have the capacity, the power, to make changes. It is important for them to see that they can be successful in making constructive modifications in their life. Successful experiences, even small successes, can help people build this sense of self-efficacy. Therefore, it is helpful to encourage people to set reasonable goals for themselves. People with sedentary lifestyles do not have to become great athletes; they simply need to increase their physical activities. Any increase should be viewed as a success. Similarly, people who have become accustomed to a diet high in fat do not have to adopt a strict, low-fat diet to be successful; they need only to reduce some of the fat in their diet to rightfully claim success. Movement in the right direction, even if it comes in small steps, can build confidence and raise expectations about their ability to make additional changes.

It is also important for people to realize that it often takes several "starts" toward a healthier lifestyle before they are able to maintain the desired changes. Many health-compromising habits are extremely hard to give up, and many health-enhancing practices are difficult to incorporate into a schedule that is already hectic and full of competing responsibilities. People should not feel bad if their initial attempts are not successful. Instead, encourage people to learn from their setbacks. For example, if they fail to maintain a regular exercise program, is it because they chose a form of exercise they do not enjoy? If so, they may want to try again, but this time choosing an activity they find pleasurable. People who are trying to give up habits such as smoking should be assured that long-term success often comes only after several attempts. Individuals who fail in their initial attempts should be commended for their efforts and encouraged to try again. Relapses should be viewed as an expected part of the lifestyle modification process and not as evidence that success will never be attained.

ON-SITE SERVICES AND SUPPORTIVE FOLLOW-UP

When planning health programs for your congregation or community, it is important to recognize the value of on-site services. Some of the steps you or your guest speakers are recommending may seem too costly, time-wise or financially, if people have to leave work or make special travel arrangements. For example, some individuals may be persuaded that it would be wise to monitor their blood pressure on a regular basis, but they find it difficult to get to their doctor's office or a clinic. Problems with transportation or scheduling may prevent them from regular visits. An easy solution to these problems is to arrange for nurses to provide blood pressure checks once a month immediately after a worship service or a regularly scheduled congregational meeting. Providing on-site services will lessen the cost or burden of following the health-enhancing recommendations people have received in your educational programs. Anything you can do to remove or reduce barriers will increase the chances of people engaging in health-enhancing activities.

Finally, the value of regular reminders and supportive follow-up services cannot be emphasized enough. People are not always ready for the information you are offering at the time you are offering it. For example, many individuals may not think they need to know much about depression the first time you provide information on mood disorders in a congregational program because it does not seem to be a factor in their life or the lives of their loved ones. However, a few months later they may be ready to hear about this topic because a family member is showing signs of depression. Now they are ready to learn more about how to recognize and respond to depression. Another reason to incorporate regular messages and reminders is that most people find it difficult to make lasting changes in their behavior patterns and health practices. Friendly reminders can help them stay on track and maintain their motivation.

3

Establishing
a Health Education Program

A congregation of almost any size can have an effective health education program. It does not need a nurse or a professional health educator on its staff to direct the program. Nor does it need to spend much money on the program. What is necessary is (1) *the initial endorsement and ongoing support of the clergy*, and (2) *the active involvement of at least one staff person or volunteer who is interested in providing leadership for the program as coordinator.* As long as these two key elements are present, you can have a significant impact on the lives of people in your congregation as well as those in the community it serves.

RESOURCES NEEDED

The resources the congregational coordinator(s) will need to run a health education program are available at little or no cost in most communities. *The first place you should go is the hospital.* Your local hospital has most of the necessary resources, and it may be interested in establishing an alliance with your congregation. We have found that many hospitals and health care professionals are interested in working with religious institutions to conduct community-based health education programs. They recognize the importance of health education and realize that they can reach many more people if they work with congregations in the community. Religious institutions generally are closer to the people than are hospitals. They are closer not only geographically but also in terms of the cultural values and traditions of their members.

We have helped many hospitals develop lay health educator programs. These programs provide training and ongoing support for volunteers from local congregations. For these programs, hospitals invite local clergy to identify "natural leaders" in their congregations who would be interested in taking the initiative in developing a health ministry. Some congregations send one volunteer, whereas others send three or four. Although a few of these volunteers have had experience in a medical field, most have had no formal training or experience in health care. These volunteers are trained and then return to their congregations to offer educational programs on health topics appropriate for their congregations and communities. Most of the training is conducted by physicians, nurses, pharmacists, social workers, and other health care professionals, many of whom also later serve as guest speakers at programs coordinated by the lay health educators in congregational or community settings.

THE PROGRAM IN ACTION

An outstanding hospital-sponsored lay health educator program is one developed by Florida Hospital, a health care system serving much of central Florida. This system, which includes hospital facilities as large as the 900-bed main hospital serving the urban Orlando community and as small as a 50-bed facility in an outlying rural community, has found that its impact on the health of the community has been greatly improved by developing partnerships with local congregations. In turn, the congregations associated with the program have found that the resources provided by the hospital have enhanced their ability to minister to their members and the surrounding community. Information on important health topics and medical services available in the community is reaching many people who previously did not have this knowledge. This program has brought together and empowered a religiously and ethnically diverse group of energetic volunteers who share a strong, genuine concern for the health and welfare of others.

Our work with the lay health educator program at Florida Hospital and at other hospitals has been tremendously gratifying. It has been rewarding to see health care professionals generously share their knowledge and energetic volunteers develop ways to pass along this knowledge to their congregations and communities. The health care professionals, lay health educators, and audiences who have participated in these programs uniformly expressed enthusiasm for their value. The volunteers who have been trained in these programs have found both satisfaction and genuine excitement in their work. The congregations that have participated have found these programs to be a revitalizing force in their lay ministry.

You may wish to talk with your hospital officials about sponsoring a lay health educator program for congregations in your community. Most community hospitals are interested in establishing community outreach programs and welcome the opportunity to work with religious institutions. If your hospital cannot take the lead in developing a lay health educator program, it still should be able to assist you in developing your own health education program. Usually there are physicians, nurses, and other health care professionals affiliated with the hospital who are eager to talk about certain health topics. Many welcome the opportunity to educate people about the steps they can take to maintain their health.

Other community institutions and national organizations can also provide resources for your program and will want to cooperate with you. Organizations such as the American Heart Association, American Cancer Society, Mental Health Association, American Geriatrics Society, and American Diabetes Association have many of the materials you will need, and they are eager to share these. In fact, they measure their success by their ability to reach people in the community. Also, some of these organizations will have a list of physicians, nurses, and other professionals who are interested in speaking at community meetings. Home health agencies are another good source of materials and speakers. We have included information about these organizations and their resources in the following chapters.

"TOP TEN" TOPICS

What topics need to be covered in a health education program? Based on interviews with physicians, nurses, social workers, clergy, and members of many religious institutions, we have assembled a "top ten" list. These subjects, some of which are not strictly medical but still relate to health, are covered in part 2 of the book. These chapters can be used in conjunction with a hospital-sponsored lay health educator program or as an outline and guide for an independently run congregational health education program. Each of the chapters follows a format that is consistent with the health belief model and that has proven useful to congregational volunteers in designing and implementing their programs. The format is as follows:

- The nature and prevalence of the disorder
- The risks of ignoring information on the disorder
- What individuals can do to prevent or reduce the impact of the disorder
- Suggestions for congregational programs
- Examples of congregational programs
- Information resources

Each of the ten topics selected has wide applicability across diverse socioeconomic, cultural, and age groups. Suggested programs focus on information and strategies that relate directly to individual health as well as the health of loved ones. Certainly our list of topics could be expanded to include many others. However, the template provided for each of the topics we selected should enable interested organizations to tailor their own programs for meeting community needs.

ESTABLISHING STANDARDS

One issue you will need to confront as you begin a congregational health education program is that of establishing standards for the topics and materials you include in your program. A visit to the health section of any bookstore will reveal why this is important. There are many books on health matters, and some of them make exaggerated or even completely unverifiable claims about the efficacy of certain treatments and practices. It is not always easy to determine which ones can be trusted. Additionally, people from your congregation or community may suggest questionable topics or speakers. One way to handle this problem is to find a physician who will serve as an advisor to your program. Ask him or her to review the topics and materials you are considering including in your program.

Another option is to adopt a book or newsletter published by a medical school as your primary reference. These publications generally take an evidence-based approach to the information and advice they offer. Their recommendations include nonmedical or "alternative medicine" interventions (e.g., exercise, nutrition, stress reduction, psychotherapy) as long as there is scientific evidence for these interventions. Although the information and recommendations provided in these books and newsletters are based on scientific research, they are written in such a manner as to be easily understood by people with no medical training.

We have chosen to rely primarily on materials published by the Johns Hopkins University School of Medicine, even though we also have had physicians from many other health care systems serving as advisors for our programs. An excellent resource is the *Johns Hopkins Family Health Book*. This is a comprehensive yet easily readable reference that offers information on available treatments and prevention. In addition to helping you establish standards by which you can make decisions about including or excluding various topics, it can serve as a valuable supplement to the medical information we provide. It offers a more extensive discussion of the symptoms and nature of each condition, and, because it includes information on all body systems, it can help you broaden the scope of your health education program beyond the topics we discuss. Another resource that has been helpful for lay health educators is *The Johns Hopkins Medical Letter Health after 50*. This newsletter is published monthly and provides valuable updates on medical topics of concern to individuals in middle to late adulthood. People who find the brief newspaper accounts of recent medical findings somewhat confusing will appreciate the more complete reports that appear in this and other newsletters published for the general public by respected medical institutions. (See the suggested readings for additional information on these publications.)

SELECTING TOPICS AND SPEAKERS FOR A CONGREGATIONAL HEALTH EDUCATION PROGRAM

When choosing topics for your health education program, especially your first few sessions, you need to be sure you select topics that are of interest to a significant number of members of your congregation. Since the concerns will vary from congregation to congregation, it is important to have a way to assess your congregation's interests. To assist in this process, we have included a sample survey (see Appendix A) that can easily be adapted for use in any congregation or group setting. It is also important to evaluate each program you offer. Participants can often provide valuable advice about what they liked (e.g., topic, speaker, format, materials) and what could be done to make the next program even better. To aid in this evaluation process, we have included a sample evaluation form (see Appendix B) that can be modified for use in congregational or community programs.

SUGGESTED TOPICS FOR
CONGREGATIONAL PROGRAMS

4

Coronary Heart Disease

Coronary heart disease is the leading cause of death in the United States. Each year approximately 1.5 million Americans suffer a heart attack and nearly half a million die as a result of the attack. Heart attacks (myocardial infarctions) occur when arterial (blood vessel) blockages stop blood and oxygen from reaching the heart muscle—as when a clogged fuel line stops a car engine. The blockage is generally due to atherosclerosis, or the build-up of plaque in the arteries. The process of plaque building up and causing a thickening or hardening of the arteries begins long before a heart attack occurs. In fact, it is a gradual process that may start as early as childhood.

The incidence of heart disease increases with age. Although heart disease is more common in men than in women during early and middle adulthood, the risk of heart disease rises dramatically in women in their fifties (after menopause). Heredity also is a significant risk factor for onset at a younger age. And, the risk of heart disease is greater if you have a family history of premature heart attacks.

THE RISKS OF IGNORING INFORMATION ON HEART DISEASE

The most serious and feared consequence of failing to heed information about heart disease is a fatal heart attack. As already mentioned, each year approximately half a million persons die as a result of a heart attack. However, what many people fail to realize is that there may be grave and long-lasting consequences for those who survive a heart attack. Congestive heart failure, most commonly caused by damaged heart muscle following

a heart attack, is a serious condition and the leading cause of hospitalization in older adults. In this condition, the heart muscle is too weak to pump
enough blood to provide the body with the oxygen it needs to meet the
demands of normal activities. The lives of people with congestive heart failure are usually seriously limited due to the fatigue and weakness associated with this condition. Even limited physical exertion can produce shortness of breath.

WHAT CAN BE DONE TO PREVENT HEART DISEASE?

Reducing the Risk of Developing Heart Disease

Many steps can be taken to avoid, or at least greatly delay, the harmful consequences of heart disease. Among the most important are changes
in lifestyle:

- *Stop smoking*. Smoking contributes to heart disease by promoting
  the build-up of plaque in the arteries. It is not easy for most people
  to stop smoking, but the benefits are significant.
- *Decrease the amount of cholesterol and saturated fat in your diet*. If
  dietary changes are not sufficient to lower cholesterol to acceptable
  levels, there are several effective medications that can be taken.
- *Exercise more often*. You do not have to embark on a rigorous and
  exhausting exercise program, but it does need to be regular.
- *Lose weight*. If you are overweight, lose weight by participating in a
  safe, gradual weight reduction program.

Another step you should consider, but only if recommended by your
physician, is taking a low dose of aspirin every day. An additional measure
women should consider and discuss with their physicians is postmeno-
pausal estrogen replacement therapy.

Detecting the Early Signs of Coronary Heart Disease

Detecting coronary heart disease can be difficult because the athero-
sclerotic process can be well advanced before there are any noticeable signs

of heart disease. For example, the pain and discomfort associated with myocardial ischemia (an inadequate flow of blood to part of the heart) may not occur until the artery is narrowed by 75 percent. This pain or discomfort is referred to as *angina pectoris* and occurs when the demand for blood and oxygen exceeds the supply. It usually follows physical activity.

Because the first signs of coronary heart disease may not occur until the arteries are already narrowed significantly, it is important for people to visit their physicians regularly or participate in cardiac screenings. The tests for cholesterol and lipoproteins are relatively simple and can be arranged through physicians' offices or hospital laboratories. If your levels are found to be high, both lifestyle modifications and medications can be used to treat the problem.

Recognizing and Reacting to Signs of a Heart Attack

Thus far we have discussed what you can do to reduce the risk of a heart attack. But what should you do if you think you or someone you are with is having a heart attack? What are the symptoms? How quickly should you react and whom should you call if you think it is a heart attack?

The steps you take during the first minutes of a suspected heart attack are extremely important. They can make the difference between life and death or long-term disability. Immediate emergency medical attention is absolutely necessary. Therefore, it is important for people to know the early signs of a heart attack. These are the warning signals:

- Chest pain—frequently described as pressure or squeezing sensations
- Pain spreading to shoulders, arms (especially the left arm), and jaw
- Sudden feeling of faintness or breathlessness
- Nausea
- Sweating

If you or a person you are with experiences these warning signs for more than a few minutes, you should call for emergency medical care immediately. Do not ignore these signs or delay getting treatment until it is more convenient.

SUGGESTIONS FOR CONGREGATIONAL PROGRAMS

- Provide assistance for members of your congregation and community who want to stop smoking. This assistance can be in the form of information on smoking cessation programs available in your community, or you may be able to arrange for classes to be offered at one of your congregation's facilities. Your hospital and the American Heart Association can give you information about programs and materials.
- Provide information on nutrition and offer samples of low-fat meals and snacks. There are several ways to do this:

  1. Have a special program on this topic, with a dietitian offering information on food selection and meal preparation.
  2. Incorporate low-fat foods into regularly scheduled congregational meals and then distribute information about the low-fat food items to those in attendance.
  3. Arrange for a dietitian to offer a series of cooking classes in which the emphasis is on the preparation of low-fat, heart-healthy meals.
  4. Have a group in the congregation prepare a book of recipes on heart-healthy meals.

  In all of these approaches, it is important to demonstrate that it is possible to have appealing, tasty meals that are also beneficial to one's health. The American Heart Association and a dietitian from the hospital can serve as valuable resources for these programs.
- Sponsor a special program on heart disease. If possible, have a physician as your guest speaker. Although a cardiologist may seem like an obvious choice as your speaker, family practitioners and internists are well prepared to speak on the subject of heart disease. This is also a good opportunity to offer blood pressure screenings and samples of low-fat foods. Often grocery stores will donate food for these programs.
- Provide assistance for people who want to participate in a program of regularly scheduled physical activity. This can be done by distributing information on exercise programs available in your commu-

nity or by sponsoring a program held in one of your congregation's facilities. Something as simple as a walking club or group that meets regularly can prove quite beneficial, and even fun, for members who wish to incorporate physical activity into their schedule. The American Heart Association can provide materials for individuals who wish to design their own exercise programs.

- Offer a workshop or class on stress management. Your hospital or a local mental health professional should be able to assist you in developing this program.

- Arrange for a cardiopulmonary resuscitation (CPR) class to be offered to members of your congregation. Encourage older adults and those who live with older adults to attend this class.

- Distribute cards describing the symptoms of a heart attack and instructions about how to respond to these symptoms. These cards can be obtained from the American Heart Association.

- Use congregational bulletins and mailings to provide members of your congregation with basic information on heart disease and regular reminders to have their blood pressure and cholesterol levels checked. Your local chapter of the American Heart Association should be able to provide you with copies of brochures and booklets for distribution to your members.

EXAMPLES OF CONGREGATIONAL PROGRAMS

An excellent special program on heart disease was held on a Saturday morning at a Catholic church. Dr. R., a member of the church, was the featured speaker for the program. Before Dr. R. spoke, those in attendance had had an opportunity to have their blood pressure checked and sample some low-fat snacks. The program then opened with the priest offering a prayer and encouraging the audience to heed the doctor's advice. Dr. R. then spoke, using a slide show prepared by the American Heart Association to illustrate his talk. The talk was followed by a question-and-answer period, a brief break during which people could talk to the doctor on a one-to-one basis, and finally a short presentation on nutrition by a speaker from the American Heart Association. Most people stayed for the entire program, and many commented on how helpful it had been.

It is not always possible to coordinate your congregation's schedule with that of physicians or other professionals. One potential solution to scheduling difficulties is the use of videotapes. Dr. S., a cardiologist who strongly believed in the value of congregational health education programs and wished to assist as much as possible, knew that he would not be able to accept all the invitations he received from congregations participating in a hospital-sponsored lay health education program. To overcome this problem, he prepared a videotape in which he spoke on hypertension and heart disease. (Videotapes on these and other health topics are available from many sources, but we have found that people prefer to hear from local physicians whom they know.)

This tape proved to be a popular and valuable part of the health education program. One African-American congregation wanted to include a presentation on heart disease and hypertension during a regularly scheduled church program. When Dr. S. was unable to attend this program, they simply brought his message to the audience of twenty-five by showing his videotape. His message was reinforced by the volunteer lay health educator who coordinated the program and the pastor, who encouraged members to follow Dr. S.'s advice. Several members of the audience responded positively to the talk, including one woman who gave a personal example of the dangers of not recognizing the symptoms of a heart attack. She related how her father had died of a heart attack a few hours after complaining of indigestion. He had failed to recognize the signs of a heart attack. She also mentioned that Dr. S.'s presentation had convinced her that she needed to resume the exercise program she had started shortly after her father's death.

INFORMATION RESOURCES

Your local chapter of the American Heart Association can provide many of the materials you will need for your programs as well as information about services and other resources in your community. These are some of the materials you will find at most American Heart Association chapters:

• Self-administered and self-scored quizzes to help people assess their knowledge of heart disease

- Brochures, slides, and videotapes describing risk factors and how to control them
- Brochures, slides, and videotapes on nutrition
- Brochures, slides, and videotapes on exercise
- Visual aids to illustrate atherosclerosis
- Posters to publicize programs and highlight important information about recognizing, preventing, and treating heart disease

The American Heart Association can also help you identify professionals, volunteers, and other organizations in your community that offer services such as the following:

- Training in CPR
- Blood pressure checks
- Smoking cessation classes and support groups
- Cholesterol level testing
- Guest speakers

During the month of February, the American Heart Association sponsors a national campaign to raise the public's awareness of heart disease. You may wish to schedule some of your programs to coincide with this national educational effort.

The American Heart Association can be reached by calling 1-800-AHAUSA1 (800-242-8721).

The following Internet Web sites have information that may be useful in your programs: < http://www.americanheart.org/ > , < http://www.nhlbi .nih.gov/nhlbi/nhlbi.htm>, and <http://www.cdc.gov/nccdphp/cardiov.htm>.

5

Hypertension

Hypertension, or high blood pressure, is generally defined as a systolic pressure of 140 mm Hg or higher or a diastolic pressure of 90 mm Hg or higher. (Some medical experts believe that lower, more inclusive limits should be used because there is evidence that the harmful effects of hypertension begin at lower ranges.) The increased pressure accelerates damage in the normally elastic arteries and, by increasing the work of the heart pumping against higher pressure, can also lead to heart failure—even in the absence of atherosclerosis.

Hypertension affects approximately 50 million Americans, but only about half know they have this condition. The prevalence of hypertension increases with age. It is estimated that approximately 60 percent of Americans aged 60 or over have hypertension. Hypertension is more common among men than women before age 55, is roughly equivalent for men and women during the next two decades, but becomes a greater risk for women after age 74. It is most common in African Americans. Obese individuals and those with a family history of hypertension also are more likely to be affected by hypertension.

THE RISKS OF IGNORING INFORMATION ON HYPERTENSION

Although hypertension frequently produces no symptoms, it can have many harmful consequences, including severe disability and death. Hypertension damages large and small arteries directly. This damage leads to disease in the tissues and organs receiving blood from the arteries. People with hypertension are at risk for stroke, heart disease, and kidney failure lead-ing to dialysis. Longstanding hypertension can initially cause the heart to hypertrophy (or become overdeveloped and thickened), resulting in re-duced pumping action, and eventually to dilate and weaken. This condition is called heart failure. Patients with heart failure tire easily and experience shortness of breath with minor exertion.

WHAT CAN BE DONE TO PREVENT HYPERTENSION?

Detecting Hypertension

Hypertension often goes undetected because it may produce no symp-toms until it seriously damages the heart, brain, or kidneys. Some people with hypertension report headaches, but generally hypertension is discov-ered during routine checks or medical examinations. Fortunately, the as-sessment of blood pressure is easy and inexpensive. The major challenge health professionals face is persuading people that they should have their blood pressure checked on a regular basis and that they should seek treat-ment if they are found to have hypertension.

Controlling Hypertension

The good news about hypertension is that many interventions can be used to prevent or treat it. Lifestyle modifications are frequently effective in preventing or controlling hypertension. These include weight loss, restric-tion of sodium, and exercise. Reduced alcohol consumption and potassium supplementation also may be useful interventions. Lifestyle modifications are generally recommended as an initial method of controlling blood pres-sure. If such modifications are insufficient to bring blood pressure under control, numerous medications can be used.

Poor compliance with recommended interventions is a significant problem in the treatment of hypertension. Studies have shown that as many as half of patients who begin treatment for hypertension fail to continue. There are many reasons for this problem. Because many people do not have any symptoms associated with their high blood pressure, they may have little motivation to continue with the lifestyle changes or medication. Some people report that they feel better when they are not taking their medication. The costs of medications may also be a deterrent to compliance. There-fore, patients need to be reminded regularly of the dangers associated with hypertension and the benefits of the treatments.

SUGGESTIONS FOR CONGREGATIONAL PROGRAMS

- Offer periodic blood pressure checks immediately before or after worship services or other congregational meetings. Active or retired nurses from your congregation should be able to provide this service. If not, hospitals and home health agencies usually can send a nurse to conduct these checks.
- Give information about locations in the community where members can have their blood pressure checked. Drugstores as well as fire stations often offer free blood pressure checks on a regular basis.
- Sponsor a special program on hypertension with a physician or nurse educator as your featured speaker. Materials for this program can be obtained from the American Heart Association.
- Sponsor a special program on antihypertensive medications with a pharmacist as your featured speaker. Encourage people to ask about their concerns. Ask the pharmacist to discuss less expensive drugs for treating hypertension, to address the economic burden of complying with prescribed regimens.
- Use congregational bulletins and mailings to provide members with basic information on hypertension. This information can be obtained from the American Heart Association. Your local chapter should be able to provide you with copies of brochures and booklets for distribution to your members.
- Use congregational bulletins and mailings to provide members with regular reminders about monitoring their blood pressure and com-plying with treatment recommendations.
- Encourage people interested in controlling hypertension to partici-pate in exercise and nutrition programs. Several suggestions for such programs are covered in chapter 4. Another suggestion for a program on nutrition and hypertension is to feature information

on sodium. One of the topics covered could be advice on how to interpret the information on sodium provided on the labels of packaged food.

EXAMPLES OF CONGREGATIONAL PROGRAMS

A successful educational program on hypertension and heart disease was coordinated by volunteers from four Protestant churches. The late afternoon program, held in the fellowship hall of one of the churches, featured a presentation by a family practice physician affiliated with the local hospital. Almost a hundred people turned out for this program. Prior to the doctor's talk, those in attendance had the opportunity to look over literature provided by the American Heart Association and have their blood pressure checked by nurses who had volunteered their time. Additionally, they were able to sample heart-healthy snacks donated by nearby grocery stores.

Dr. C., an enthusiastic and entertaining speaker, provided the audience with a good description of hypertension, the dangers associated with ignoring this condition, and the approaches generally recommended for its treatment. He spent half an hour talking about hypertension and then took questions from the audience for another half an hour. Many people asked questions, and several questions revealed that there were a lot of misconceptions about hypertension. By the end of the hour, it was clear that the program had succeeded in alerting the audience to the serious consequences of untreated hypertension and the need for adults to have their blood pressure checked on a regular basis. The program also succeeded in correcting some of the common misunderstandings about hypertension and its treatment.

Another successful program on hypertension was organized by volunteers from three African-American Protestant congregations. They felt that many people in their congregations were unaware of the dangers of untreated hypertension and needed a better understanding of this condition. The volunteers invited Dr. S., a cardiologist associated with the hospital where most members of the congregations received their medical care, to be the guest speaker at the Friday evening program. They also arranged to have volunteer nurses available to conduct blood pressure checks and distribute materials provided by the American Heart Association. More than forty persons attended this program. Dr. S. opened his presentation with an enthusiastic endorsement of the role churches can play in the health of their members and then proceeded to describe the basic nature of hypertension, explain why it increases the risk of heart attack and stroke, and offer information about the treatments available. The audience responded well to his presentation. Several questions were asked, and a few in the audience commented that they were going to encourage family members and friends to have their blood pressure checked. Following Dr. S.'s presentation, the audience was invited to sample some of the heart-healthy snacks that the volunteers had prepared.

INFORMATION RESOURCES

Your local chapter of the American Heart Association can provide many of the materials you will need for your programs as well as information about services and other resources in your community. These are some of the materials you will find at most American Heart Association chapters:

- Brochures, slides, and videotapes describing risk factors for hypertension and how to control them
- Brochures, slides, and videotapes on nutrition and hypertension
- Brochures, slides, and videotapes on exercise and hypertension
- Posters to publicize programs and highlight important information about recognizing, preventing, and treating hypertension
- Wallet cards with tips on hypertension and a blood pressure and weight record

The American Heart Association can also help you identify professionals, volunteers, and other organizations in your community that offer services such as the following:

- Blood pressure checks
- Smoking cessation classes and support groups
- Stroke rehabilitation programs

The American Heart Association can be reached by calling 1-800-AHAUSA1 (800-242-8721).

The following Internet Web sites have information that may be useful in your programs: <http://www.americanheart.org/>, <http://www.nhlbi.nih.gov/nhlbi/nhlbi.htm>, and <http://www.stroke.org/>.

6

Cancer

There are more than 100 types of cancer, all characterized by the uncontrolled growth and spread of abnormal cells. The most common types are prostate, breast, lung, and colon cancer, each of which typically begins as a discrete localized tumor (or mass) in the affected organ. (Some less common cancers of the bloodstream, such as lymphoma or leukemia, involve the body more generally at the time of presentation.) Initially, most cancers are generally localized, with cancer cells confined to their original site. Later, cancer cells may spread or metastasize to other sites. Treatment is more successful when cancer is localized; once cancer cells have spread, treatment is more difficult and less effective.

More than 1,200,000 new cases of cancer are diagnosed each year. Approximately 550,000 Americans die from cancer each year, making it the second leading cause of death in the United States.

The incidence and mortality rates for cancer are generally higher for African Americans than for Caucasians. Also, the five-year survival rate for cancer in African Americans is significantly lower, due in large part to late diagnoses.

THE RISKS OF IGNORING INFORMATION ON CANCER

Fear and fatalism often interfere with people obtaining accurate information about cancer and the appropriate tests and treatment options. Many individuals are so fearful of cancer that they do not want to know much about it or participate in screenings that might detect it. Often their fear is combined with a fatalistic view of cancer; they believe that there is little they can do to prevent it and that there are virtually no effective treatments. People need help in overcoming their fear and sense of hopelessness about cancer. In recent years, screening for cancer has become more precise, and early detection has reduced some cancer death rates. People need to know that not only are there steps they can take to reduce their risk of developing cancer but also that other steps can result in early detection and cure.

WHAT CAN BE DONE TO PREVENT CANCER?

It is extremely important for cancer to be detected and treated as early as possible. Generally, the earlier the treatment begins, the better the chance of curing or controlling the cancer. The overall survival rate for many cancers would increase significantly if more people would participate in early detection programs. A combination of regular self-exams and screenings provides the best means of detecting cancer early enough to allow for effective treatment. Unfortunately, too many people ignore the recommendations about regular self-exams and screenings.

The National Cancer Institute recommends using the mnemonic C-A-U-T-I-O-N as an outline for recognizing common warning signs of cancer:

Change in bowel or bladder habits
A sore that does not heal
Unusual bleeding or discharge
Thickening or lump in the breast or elsewhere
Indigestion or difficulty swallowing
Obvious change in wart or mole
Nagging cough or hoarseness

These signs and symptoms are not definite indicators of cancer; they can be caused by other problems. However, if they persist for more than two weeks, it is wise to see a physician.

People also need to be aware that their risk of developing cancer can be reduced by making modifications in their lifestyle. Most important is smoking cessation. The American Cancer Society estimates that more than

80 percent of lung cancer deaths result from smoking and that almost 175,000 cancer deaths each year can be attributed to the use of tobacco. However, even longtime smokers who quit have a reduced risk (compared with people who continue smoking) of lung, laryngeal, esophageal, oral, pancreatic, bladder, and cervical cancer.

Diet can play an important role in reducing the incidence of cancer. High-fat or low-fiber diets may play a causative role in cancer, whereas the daily consumption of vegetables and fruits is associated with a lower risk of lung, prostate, bladder, esophageal, and stomach cancers.

Often people do not realize that the chance of getting cancer increases with age. For example, breast cancer is thought by many to be a disease that primarily affects middle-aged women; in fact, the incidence of breast cancer rises steadily with age. Therefore, it is important for older women to have regular physical examinations and mammograms.

A special effort needs to be made to encourage minorities to participate in early detection programs. Their lower rates of participation have resulted in later detection of cancers and higher mortality rates. In addition, some people fail to participate in regular screenings for cancer because of their fear of the pain or indignities associated with the screenings. Therefore, accurate information about the nature of the screenings and the definite benefits of early detection needs to be provided.

Many people believe that there are no effective treatments for most types of cancer or that the available treatments are worse than the disease. Consequently, it is important that they be given honest, accurate information about treatments and their right to choose treatments. Patients should be encouraged to ask their physicians about treatment options, the risks and side effects as well as the expected benefits of the treatments, and the likely consequences of no treatment.

Support groups can be quite helpful to those with cancer. They can provide valuable emotional support, and there is evidence that cancer patients who participate in support groups live longer.

SUGGESTIONS FOR CONGREGATIONAL PROGRAMS

- Arrange for cancer screenings. Some hospitals have mobile mammography units that can be sent to your community. If such a unit is not available, you may be able to arrange transportation to the local hospital for members of your congregation. Screenings for colorectal cancer and skin cancer are also advised. Check with the hospital to find out the easiest way to provide these screenings for members of your congregation and community.

- Provide help for members of your congregation and community who want to stop smoking. You could inform them about smoking cessation programs offered in your community, or you could sponsor a class held in one of your congregation's facilities. You can obtain information about programs and materials from the local hospital and the American Cancer Society.
- Distribute materials to specific groups within your congregation. For example, give information on breast cancer to women's groups and information on prostate cancer to men's groups. Printed materials and videotapes from the American Cancer Society are available.
- Distribute information on skin cancer and sun exposure to all age groups, but make a special effort to reach children, teenagers, and young adults in the congregation. You may wish to emphasize this topic during the spring and summer months.
- Sponsor a special program on cancer. An oncologist or medical professional who is regularly involved in the diagnosis or treatment of cancer can serve as your featured speaker. The American Cancer Society can provide you with materials to distribute at this program.
- Sponsor or help members of your congregation find a support group for people who have cancer. Potential leaders for a support group include hospital social workers, mental health professionals, nurses, and cancer survivors. The hospital and the American Cancer Society can help you locate existing groups or identify qualified group leaders.

EXAMPLES OF CONGREGATIONAL PROGRAMS

An excellent congregational program on cancer was coordinated by a lay health educator from a Protestant church. She asked Dr. M., the oncologist who had spoken to her lay health educator class, to speak to members of her congregation about cancer. She specifically requested that the doctor address the nature of cancer, how to prevent it, and how to treat it. Dr. M. opened with a general overview of cancer, then focused on breast cancer for the remainder of her presentation. She used slides to illustrate some of the breast cancers she has treated. The slides were disturbing, but Dr. M., the lay health educator, and the minister had agreed in advance that the audience needed to see these pictures. The doctor's presentation, including the slides, clearly held the people's interest. The many questions asked by the audience provided evidence of the high level of interest in the topic of cancer. Additionally, most of the people in the audience picked up some of the American Cancer Society materials that had been brought to the meeting by the lay health educator, and many took the time to thank her for arranging this presentation.

Another good health education program on cancer, which was targeted at a specific group—those at risk for prostate cancer—was held at an African-American church. The lay health educator, a registered nurse at a community hospital, arranged for an African-American physician who worked at her hospital to speak at a regularly scheduled meeting of the men of the church. After introducing the doctor, the lay health educator excused herself from the meeting, leaving only the men in the room. The doctor gave a brief talk on prostate cancer and then answered questions from the audience. Many of the men who attended this meeting reported that it had been very informative and that they intended to follow the doctor's recommendations.

INFORMATION RESOURCES

Your local chapter of the American Cancer Society can provide many of the materials you will need for your programs as well as information about services and other resources in your community. These are some of the materials you will find at most American Cancer Society chapters:

- Self-administered and self-scored quizzes to help people assess their knowledge of risk factors for cancer
- Brochures, fact sheets, and videotapes describing risk factors and how to control them

- Brochures, fact sheets, and videotapes on various types of cancer
- Brochures, fact sheets, and videotapes on cancer designed for specific groups (e.g., men, women, African Americans)
- Brochures describing and illustrating self-examinations
- Posters to publicize programs and highlight important information about recognizing, preventing, and treating cancer
- Brochures on healthy diet

The American Cancer Society can also help you identify professionals, volunteers, and other organizations in your community that can offer services such as the following:

- Guest speakers for community programs
- Support groups for cancer patients and families
- Trained cancer survivors who can offer support and information for patients
- Assistance with transportation and supplies
- Smoking cessation classes

The American Cancer Society sponsors public awareness campaigns throughout the year. The society can be reached by calling 1-800-ACS-2345 (800-227-2345).

The following Internet Web sites provide information on cancer: <http://www.cancer.org/>, <http://www.cdc.gov/nccdphp/cancer.htm>, and <http://www.nci.nih.gov/>.

7

Diabetes Mellitus

It is estimated that more than 16 million Americans have diabetes mellitus, a condition defined by abnormally high blood levels of glucose (a natural sugar). However, only about half of the individuals who have diabetes have been diagnosed. Among people 65 years of age and older, it is estimated that 15 to 20 percent have diabetes mellitus. The prevalence rates are even higher among African Americans and Mexican Americans, and for all adults who are overweight.

There are two types of diabetes mellitus. *Type I* diabetes mellitus, also known as insulin-dependent diabetes mellitus, juvenile diabetes, and brittle diabetes, accounts for approximately 10 percent of all cases. This type is most likely to affect those under the age of 20, although it can occur at older ages. More common is *type II* diabetes mellitus, also referred to as noninsulin-dependent diabetes mellitus or adult-onset diabetes, generally found in individuals over the age of 40. Type II diabetes accounts for approximately 90 percent of all cases. Although the majority of type II diabetics are overweight, even lean adults can be affected.

In diabetic persons, high blood glucose (hyperglycemia) occurs because there is a breakdown in the normal process of glucose being transported into the body's cells. Insulin, a hormone produced by the pancreas, plays a critical role in the transportation of glucose into the cells. High levels of blood glucose result when there is not enough insulin produced by the pancreas (type I diabetes) or when the cells are resistant or unresponsive to insulin (type II diabetes).

Type I diabetes usually develops rapidly, with individuals experiencing unexplained weight loss, frequent urination, and excessive thirst. Sometimes diabetic ketoacidosis, a potentially life-threatening condition with symptoms that include nausea, vomiting, slow respirations, and mental confusion, can be the presenting illness for type I diabetics. Type II diabetes develops more gradually, with many individuals experiencing few or no symptoms for several years. Increased thirst and urination can be seen along with visual disturbances or even fungal rashes of the feet or groin. Occasionally individuals with type II diabetes suffer ketoacidosis under certain circumstances, but the more serious problems associated with type II diabetes are its long-term complications.

THE RISKS OF IGNORING INFORMATION ON DIABETES

The millions of people who have diabetes but who are not receiving treatment are at risk for many of the chronic complications of diabetes. Undetected and untreated diabetes sets the stage for other diseases or conditions that can kill or cripple:

- *Stroke*: Older adults with diabetes are almost twice as likely as those without diabetes to have a stroke.
- *Heart disease*: Older adults with diabetes are twice as likely to develop cardiovascular disease, and heart attacks are more likely to be fatal.
- *Amputation*: The risk of lower-extremity amputation is ten times greater for older adults with diabetes.
- *Eye disease*: Cataracts, glaucoma, and retinopathy (damage to the retina) are more common among older adults with diabetes.
- *Kidney disease*: Approximately 20 percent of individuals with type II diabetes develop nephropathy (kidney damage) that often leads to kidney failure and the need for dialysis.

WHAT CAN BE DONE TO PREVENT DIABETES?

If diabetes is detected and treated aggressively, some of the long-term complications can be eliminated or their severity greatly reduced. However, many adults are unaware that they have diabetes until they are treated for one of the chronic complications. Therefore, it is important to persuade people to have regular medical examinations, even if they are feeling well. Diabetes is usually diagnosed based on blood tests in which abnormally high glucose levels are found.

Although treatment for type I diabetes includes daily injections of insulin, many cases of type II diabetes do not require insulin injections. Type II diabetes often can be controlled through diet, weight control, and exercise. Oral hypoglycemic drugs may be needed if diet and exercise do not adequately control glucose levels.

Although it may seem that people who are diagnosed with type II diabetes have a relatively simple treatment regimen to follow, the fact is that many find it difficult to follow their doctor's recommendations consistently. It is not easy to make major lifestyle changes, especially when there are no immediately noticeable consequences. Changes in established patterns are difficult to make and even more difficult to maintain. Therefore, patients need the ongoing encouragement and support of family and friends.

SUGGESTIONS FOR CONGREGATIONAL PROGRAMS

- Sponsor glucose level testing by working with representatives from the local hospital's medical laboratory or another community medical laboratory. If these representatives cannot conduct the testing at your facility, perhaps you can arrange for transportation to their facility.
- Sponsor a special program on diabetes with a physician, nurse educator, or dietitian as your featured speaker. Provide snacks appropriate for people with diabetes.
- Sponsor a support group for patients and families affected by diabetes. Support groups can assist patients in complying with treatment recommendations and also in coping with some of the emotional challenges often associated with diabetes. Your hospital or the American Diabetes Association can assist you in establishing a support group or in locating support groups in the community.
- Sponsor or help members of your congregation locate exercise and weight reduction programs. Most people find it easier to sustain their exercise or weight reduction efforts if they are a part of a group.
- Sponsor cooking classes for patients and families affected by dia-

betes. A hospital dietitian or the American Diabetes Association can assist with materials and other resources for this program.

- Use congregational bulletins and mailings to provide members with basic information on diabetes. This information can be obtained from many sources, including materials available from the American Diabetes Association. Your local chapter should be able to provide copies of brochures and booklets for distribution to your members.
- Use church bulletins and mailings to provide members with regular reminders about monitoring their glucose level and complying with treatment recommendations.

EXAMPLES OF CONGREGATIONAL PROGRAMS

A congregational health education program on diabetes held at a Protestant church illustrates many features of an effective health ministry. An active church volunteer who had participated in a hospital-sponsored lay health educator training program offered to coordinate a series of five programs on various health issues. She and her minister decided they should offer the series at the beginning of the new year because that is when many people resolve to make improvements in their lives. The series was introduced at the first worship service of the year by the senior minister, who preached a sermon entitled "A Theology of Health." Building on the theme of stewardship of the body, he encouraged members of the congregation to join him in making a commitment to improve their health. The first workshop was scheduled for that Sunday evening, with subsequent workshops held on Wednesday evenings following the regularly scheduled church supper.

The workshop on diabetes, held in the chapel on a Wednesday evening, drew an overflow crowd of more than a hundred people. The size of the audience was the result of several factors: The program had been announced in the Sunday worship services, a written announcement was placed in the church bulletin, and the senior minister had urged people present at the dinner to attend the workshop.

The featured speaker was Dr. N., a physician well known in the community not only for his work with diabetes but also his enthusiasm and speaking ability. Also, it was clear that the strong endorsements offered by the minister and the respected church volunteer added credibility to the doctor's presentation. Dr. N. gave a brief description of the two types of diabetes, talked about the large number of people who have diabetes but are not yet symptomatic, listed the dangerous health consequences of failing to detect and treat diabetes, and offered information on the different approaches to the treatment of diabetes. Although some of his talk was disturbing, his overall message was encouraging—people can maintain their health if they have a good understanding of their medical condition and follow the recommendations of a trusted physician.

A Seventh-Day Adventist church conducted screenings for diabetes during a health fair held at the church. The health fair was announced to members of the congregation in the church bulletin and at the worship service. The church also publicized the fair in the surrounding community by hanging a banner near the church's street and placing announcements in a neighborhood newspaper. The lay health educator arranged for a representative from the local hospital to conduct the screenings. The hospital representative brought a blood glucose meter and all the other necessary materials. Because the test required only a drop of blood taken from a finger and could be completed in a couple of minutes, dozens of people were able to be screened. The lay health educator who coordinated the health fair reported two particularly significant findings. First, a Haitian woman was found to have a blood sugar level of 300. She told the attending nurse that she had been feeling sick. She also reported experiencing increased thirst and urination, symptoms associated with diabetes. With the assistance and encouragement of the nurse, the woman immediately went to a nearby medical clinic for further testing and treatment. Second, a man tested with an elevated blood sugar level. When the nurse informed him, the man acknowledged that he had been diagnosed with diabetes but had failed to comply with his doctor's treatment recommendations. The nurse explained the dangers of failing to control diabetes and referred the man back to his doctor, strongly encouraging him to follow the medical advice he had been given.

INFORMATION RESOURCES

Your local chapter of the American Diabetes Association can provide many of the materials you will need for your programs as well as information about services and other resources in your community. These are some of the materials you will find at most American Diabetes Association chapters:

- Self-administered and self-scored quizzes to help people assess their risk of diabetes
- Brochures and fact sheets describing the dangers of undetected and untreated diabetes
- Brochures and fact sheets designed for specific groups (e.g., African Americans, Hispanics)
- Nutrition guides for people with diabetes
- Posters to publicize programs and highlight important information about diabetes
- Self-care guides, cookbooks and meal planners, and medical management guidelines

The American Diabetes Association can also help you identify professionals, volunteers, and other organizations in your community that offer services such as the following:

- Guest speakers for congregational and community programs
- Support groups for patients with diabetes and their families
- Educational classes (e.g., nutrition) for patients with diabetes and their families
- Information on medical supplies

The American Diabetes Association sponsors a national diabetes awareness campaign every November. You may wish to schedule a congregational program on diabetes to coincide with this national campaign. The American Diabetes Association can be reached by calling 1-800-DIABETES (800-342-2383).

The following Internet Web sites provide information on diabetes: <http://www.diabetes.org/>, <http://www.niddk.nih.gov/>, and <http://www.cdc.gov/nccdphp/ddt/ddthome.htm>.

8

Depression

Depression, a serious condition that affects millions of Americans every year, is different from the periods of sadness or feelings of grief that occur as an expected part of life for most people. Although it is normal to be sad or "down" occasionally and to experience grief when a significant loss occurs, clinical depression has more severe symptoms and is more likely to affect an individual's ability to function normally.

It is estimated that during any given month, almost 5 percent of Americans will experience an episode of major depression. The lifetime prevalence of major depression is more than 17 percent. When other depressive disorders (i.e., bipolar disorder, dysthymic disorder) are included, the estimate of lifetime prevalence exceeds 20 percent. In other words, one of every five Americans will experience at least one serious episode of depression at some point during his or her lifetime. Females are approximately twice as likely as males to experience an episode of major depression. Recent studies indicate that depression is increasing among the young, with younger age cohorts more likely to experience depression than older ones.

Depression is not only a painful condition but also one that can greatly impair a person's relationships and ability to work productively. In many cases it is a life-threatening condition, placing people at risk for death from suicide or physical conditions such as heart disease.

One of the most unfortunate and tragic aspects of depression is that in spite of the availability of several effective methods of treatment, it frequently goes undetected and untreated. Often the symptoms are incorrectly attributed to medical conditions or other factors (e.g., aging). Even when people are aware of their depression, they may underestimate the seriousness of the disorder or feel hopeless about finding effective treatment. Many people, especially elderly individuals, do not view depression as a serious condition that may require professional help; they believe that they are responsible for bringing on the depression and that only they can "remove" their depression.

Because depression is so frequently undetected, it is important for congregational health education programs to inform their members about the symptoms of depression. These are the most common symptoms:

- Depressed mood with overwhelming feelings of sadness and grief
- Loss of interest and pleasure in activities formerly enjoyed
- Insomnia, early morning waking, or oversleeping nearly every day
- Decreased energy; fatigue
- Noticeable changes in appetite and weight (a significant loss or gain)
- Feelings of guilt, worthlessness, and helplessness
- Inability to concentrate or think; indecisiveness
- Recurrent thoughts of death and suicide
- Restlessness or slowing down

An episode of major depression is diagnosed when a person has experienced five or more of these symptoms every day or almost every day during a two-week period. At least one of the symptoms must be depressed mood or loss of interest or pleasure in activities previously enjoyed.

Another form of depression is dysthymic disorder. This is a milder but chronic pattern of depression. People with this disorder experience symptoms of depression almost every day for at least two years. During this period, they are never without the symptoms of depression for more than two months. In addition to depressed mood, they experience two or more of the following symptoms:

- Poor appetite or overeating
- Insomnia or hypersomnia
- Low energy or fatigue
- Low self-esteem
- Poor concentration or difficulty making decisions
- Feelings of hopelessness

A third mood disorder in which a person experiences episodes of depression is bipolar disorder (also known as manic-depressive disorder). In addition to the depression, the person also experiences mania or hypomania. Symptoms of mania or hypomania are as follows:

- Inflated self-esteem or grandiosity
- Decreased need for sleep
- Unusual need to talk more or feelings of pressure to keep talking
- Flight of ideas or subjective experience that thoughts are racing
- Distractibility
- Increase in goal-directed activity or psychomotor agitation
- Excessive involvement in pleasurable activities that have a high potential for painful consequences

In the case of a manic episode, at least three of these symptoms persist for at least one week and are severe enough to impair significantly occupational or social functioning. In the case of hypomania, the symptoms persist for at least four days but do not significantly impair occupational or social functioning.

The primary reason that it is important to note whether a depression is accompanied by symptoms of mania or hypomania is that bipolar disorders require different treatment from what is typically used for unipolar depressions (i.e., major depression and dysthymic disorder).

THE RISKS OF IGNORING INFORMATION ON DEPRESSION

The most serious consequence of failing to detect and treat depression is the greatly increased risk of suicide. The suicide rate increases with age and is highest among older men. The tremendous emotional pain, combined with the sense of hopelessness about ever obtaining relief from the pain, leads many depressed people to see death as their only escape.

Because of the harmful effects of depression on the immune system and the feelings of hopelessness and helplessness associated with depression, depressed people are more likely to experience other health problems and suffer more harmful consequences from existing physical illnesses. For example, someone who suffers a heart attack and is depressed is more likely to die than someone who suffers a heart attack but is not depressed. In addition, depressed people are less likely to follow the treatment recommendations for their other conditions and diseases.

The emotional and financial costs of depression often go well beyond the depressed person. Depression can contribute to marital and family conflict, work impairment, and financial problems. Too frequently we read accounts in the newspaper of destructive or deadly actions that were caused at least in part by depression.

WHAT CAN BE DONE TO PREVENT DEPRESSION?

The first step that needs to be taken in any congregational program on depression is to increase the members' ability to recognize this disorder. Depression often goes undetected because we attribute some of the symptoms to other factors. For example, we may not be surprised when a teenager seems moody and withdraws from family and friends. We may assume that this is typical and does not call for any special attention. Depression can also be especially difficult to detect among the elderly. Older adults are less likely to report that they are depressed, and often the symptoms of depression are attributed to physical disorders or are thought to be a normal part of aging. Because of these difficulties in detecting depression, a health education program needs to find creative ways to distribute information about the symptoms of depression. People need to be able to recognize the symptoms of depression in themselves and others.

The second step is to give people hope about the treatment for depression. There are several effective biological and psychological treatments for depression. People with depression are not doomed to a life of misery if they seek professional help, but many fail to ask for help. Why? One reason is the stigma that many people still feel is attached to depression or any mental disorder. They believe that it is a sign of weakness or moral failure. Many believe that if their faith were only stronger they would not be depressed. Because of these beliefs, they are embarrassed to let others know they are depressed. These beliefs can constitute a serious and dangerous barrier to treatment. A congregational health education program must find ways to knock down this barrier.

The third step is to give the congregation reliable, up-to-date information on treatment options. They should learn about both biological and psychological methods. Currently, many excellent medications are available. The antidepressant medications that have been around the longest (e.g., Pamelor and Norpramin) are still recognized as effective in relieving depression, but the newer ones (e.g., Zoloft, Paxil, and Prozac) are also effective and have fewer side effects. This is an important consideration because many people stop taking medications if they produce unpleasant side effects. Antidepressant medication should result in significant improvement within six weeks. Most of these medications can be prescribed by a family physician.

Most of the psychological therapies that have been demonstrated to be effective in the treatment of depression are relatively short term and focused. They do not involve years of treatment or a detailed examination of childhood issues. In fact, psychotherapy should produce noticeable improvement within six weeks. Psychological treatment in combination with antidepressant medication is especially effective in relieving depression.

Electroconvulsive therapy (ECT) has been demonstrated to be an effective treatment for certain types of severe depression that do not respond to other forms of treatment. ECT is not the barbaric treatment it once appeared to be. Patients do not experience pain during the treatments, and their bodies do not shake or jerk. Although there may be short-term confusion after each treatment, there are seldom any signs of memory problems two to three weeks after the treatments are completed.

The fourth step is to inform the congregation about the risk of suicide among those suffering from depression. Suicides occur among all age groups, but suicide rates are highest among older adults, especially males. Often these suicides are related to a personal or family illness. Among teenagers, suicide is one of the leading killers, and recent studies show an increase in the number of suicides for the 5–19 age group. Suicides among teenagers and young adults are frequently linked to problems in relationships.

Finally, the congregational program on depression should provide guidance and support for individuals who have loved ones who are depressed. It can be especially challenging to try to care for persons who no longer find pleasure in any of the activities they previously enjoyed and who are thoroughly pessimistic about ever feeling better. The National Institute of Mental Health (NIMH) offers the following suggestions for families and friends:

- Encourage the depressed person to get appropriate treatment.
- Maintain as normal a relationship as possible.
- Point out distorted negative thinking without being critical or disapproving.
- Acknowledge that the person is suffering and in pain.
- Offer kind words and pay compliments.
- Express affection.
- Show that you care, respect, and value the depressed person.
- Do not blame the depressed person for his or her condition.
- Do not criticize, pick on, "put down," or voice disapproval until the depressed person is feeling better.
- Do not say or do anything to exacerbate the depressed person's poor self-image.

SUGGESTIONS FOR CONGREGATIONAL PROGRAMS

- Raise your congregation's awareness of depression by placing information on the symptoms, prevalence, and treatment of depression in congregational bulletins and mailings. Special attention should be given to the encouraging news about effective treatments for depression. Materials on these topics can be obtained from the Mental Health Association, the NIMH, and the Depressive and Manic Depressive Association.
- Reduce the stigma attached to depression by having respected leaders of your congregation emphasize that depression is a common disorder that does not reflect weakness or moral failure. It should be recognized and treated as a medical condition, not as a character flaw. The personal testimony of an individual who has experienced depression and knows the definite benefits of medical and psychological treatments can be especially effective.
- Provide members of your congregation with information about support groups and other services available to people encountering stressful experiences (e.g., marital separation or divorce, chronic illnesses). If there are no support groups in your community, your congregation may wish to help organize and sponsor one.
- Sponsor a class on pain management for individuals experiencing

chronic pain. Physicians and psychologists who specialize in pain management can teach strategies and skills that can help people reduce their pain and give them greater independence. Your hospital or an agency specializing in rehabilitation medicine should be able to help you locate a professional to teach the class.

- Offer a special program on antidepressant medications. A physician or pharmacist can provide information that can allay some of the fears and correct misconceptions about these medications. One specific issue that should be addressed is the need for people to take the medications as prescribed. Too often patients fail to understand and follow doctors' recommendations.

- Incorporate information on depression into regularly scheduled programs and activities. Many of the people who need information on depression may be reluctant to attend a special program on the subject. They may feel more comfortable if this information is provided in regularly scheduled programs.

- Arrange for a mental health professional to provide training for congregational leaders who teach classes or who have responsibility for visiting members so that these individuals can learn how to check for symptoms of depression. This will enable the leaders to determine whether members who decrease their participation in congregational activities they previously enjoyed could be suffering from depression.

- Find opportunities for discussions on suicide among the various age groups in your congregation. This topic needs to be addressed openly. People need to learn that the hopelessness expressed by depressed persons often leads to suicide.

- Publish in congregational bulletins and mailings the telephone numbers of the local suicide hotline and other agencies where a person in distress can call or visit if he or she needs immediate assistance.

- Encourage people to read first-person accounts to obtain a better understanding of the depressive experience and help them see that even intelligent, successful people can suffer from depression. Three books that can be recommended are *Darkness Visible*, by William Styron; *Undercurrents*, by Martha Manning, Ph.D.; and *An*

Unquiet Mind, by Kay Redfield Jamison, Ph.D. Additional information on these books is provided under the suggested readings section.

EXAMPLES OF CONGREGATIONAL PROGRAMS

An effective congregational program on depression took place one Friday evening in the Shabbat service at a Jewish temple. Midway through the service, the rabbi introduced Dr. H., a psychiatrist, who spoke for about fifteen minutes on many important aspects of depression. He described the symptoms, causal factors, and some of the treatments that are available. He pointed out that depression is a treatable disorder, but that often persons suffering from depression feel so hopeless and helpless that they fail to realize there are effective treatments available. He also pointed out that family members and friends frequently fail to detect the signs of depression, or they attribute them to other causes. Dr. H. emphasized the great importance of recognizing and treating depression because untreated depression may lead to suicide. At the conclusion of the presentation, the rabbi joined him and encouraged members of the congregation to ask questions about depression and other mental disorders. After a few questions, the rabbi invited others who had questions to speak with Dr. H. at the Oneg that followed the service. Several members of the congregation did use this opportunity to speak with him about personal concerns.

A program on depression that was offered to a group of visually impaired persons who met regularly at a community church showed how a congregational health ministry can reach out to other groups in the community. Dr. D., a clinical psychologist with a strong interest in the subject of depression, was invited to speak to the group. He gave the group a broad overview of depression and suicide, and then offered to answer questions. The responses of the audience indicated that there was considerable interest in these subjects. Many of those in attendance reported that they had experienced depression or knew someone close to them who had been depressed. They were eager to learn more about how to cope with depression and how to respond to others who seemed depressed and perhaps suicidal. The questions and comments revealed misunderstandings about antidepressant medications, and Dr. D. provided the correct information on these medications (e.g., how long it takes for a patient to respond to medication, which in some cases may be several weeks).

INFORMATION RESOURCES

Your local chapter of the Mental Health Association can provide many of the materials you can use in your programs as well as information about other resources in your community. These are some of the materials you will find at most Mental Health Association offices:

- Brochures and fact sheets on depression and other mental disorders
- Lists of symptoms designed to help people recognize depression
- Brochures and fact sheets on treatments for depression
- Brochures and fact sheets designed to reduce the stigma of depression and other mental disorders

The Mental Health Association can also help you identify professionals, volunteers, and other organizations in your community that offer services such as the following:

- Guest speakers for community programs
- Support groups for depressed persons and their families
- Support groups for persons going through various stressful experiences
- Screenings and referrals

If you have trouble locating your local chapter or need additional materials, you can call the National Mental Health Association at 1-800-969-NMHA (800-969-6642).

Materials on depression can be ordered through the DEPRESSION Awareness, Recognition, and Treatment (D/ART) Program sponsored by the NIMH (1-800-421-4211). The National Depressive and Manic Depressive Association also has materials appropriate for use in congregational programs and can be called at 1-800-82-NDMDA (800-826-3632).

The following Internet Web sites provide information on depression: <http://www.nmha.org/>, <http://www.nimh.nih.gov/>, <http://www.nami .org/>, and <http://www.ndmda.org/>. In addition, information on depression and other mental disorders can be found in *Helping Someone with Mental Illness*, by Rosalynn Carter (see the suggested readings).

9

Dementia

Dementia is a clinical syndrome or condition in which there is a progressive deterioration of mental faculties. Problems with memory are usually the first sign of dementia. Other symptoms may include difficulties with language, impaired judgment, problems in performing simple tasks such as dressing, and changes in personality and behavior.

Dementia is not an inevitable consequence of aging. Although the risk of dementia increases with age, the overwhelming majority of older adults do not have dementia. It is important to understand that most older adults who report problems with memory do not have and will not develop dementia. Minor problems with memory may be a normal part of aging and should not be viewed as evidence of dementia.

Dementia can be caused by a number of brain disorders. The most common dementia is Alzheimer disease, which accounts for approximately 50 to 60 percent of all cases of dementia. This is a progressive, degenerative disease that attacks the brain. There is loss of nerve cells, especially in the regions responsible for memory and intellectual functions. Currently there is no cure for this irreversible disease, although several newer medications can result in modest improvements in mental functions for some affected people.

Dementia resulting from vascular disease is the second most common type of dementia. This form of dementia occurs when there is damage to multiple small areas of the brain. This is typically thought to arise as a series of "small strokes" resulting from atherosclerosis and blockage of small arteries in the brain that occur over a period of months or years. For this reason, vascular dementia is now generally referred to as *multi-infarct dementia*. There are many risk factors for vascular dementia; the most important is hypertension. Individuals can reduce their risk of experiencing this form of dementia by controlling their blood pressure, avoiding smoking, eating a low-fat diet, exercising regularly, and controlling their weight.

Sometimes other conditions are mistaken for dementia. These are often referred to as *pseudodementias*. The most common condition that simulates dementia is depression. Depressed individuals may have problems with memory, experience periods of confusion, and be unresponsive to other people. It is important to distinguish correctly between depression and dementia because there are effective medical and psychological treatments for depression. Other causes of pseudodementias include overmedication, unusual drug reactions, thyroid disease, and some vitamin deficiencies. Like depression, these can be treated if they are correctly identified.

THE RISKS OF IGNORING INFORMATION ON DEMENTIA

The potential harm of relying on inaccurate or incomplete information about dementia and the health care resources appropriate for managing this condition goes far beyond the patient. Dementia is frequently referred to as a "caregiver's disease" because of its tremendous impact on the family. The spouse and other members of the patient's family face many new challenges and stresses that can seem overwhelming and endless. The decisions and pressures the family faces may produce conflict among family members. Also, it is not uncommon for family members to experience depression in reaction to this difficult situation. Family members who confront these challenges without the appropriate knowledge, skills, and resources are in danger of developing their own health problems.

The belief that dementia is inevitable and that there is no effective treatment for any type of dementia can have painful consequences for patients and their families. Patients who are thought to have dementia but who actually are depressed suffer unnecessary pain and limitations, and so do their families.

In addition, the belief that nothing that can be done to prevent the development of dementia can have harmful consequences. This belief, frequently based on the mistaken notion that all dementias are the result of Alzheimer disease, can become a self-fulfilling prophecy. In fact, several steps can be taken to reduce the risk of experiencing vascular dementia. Furthermore, these same steps may also reduce the risk of developing the symptoms of Alzheimer disease. Recent studies have shown that some people with the brain abnormalities associated with Alzheimer disease do not show its symptoms. Researchers found that it is the combination of the brain deterioration of Alzheimer disease and one or more small strokes in certain regions of the brain that most likely results in the memory loss and confusion associated with Alzheimer disease.

WHAT CAN BE DONE TO REDUCE THE IMPACT OF DEMENTIA?

Although there is no cure for most cases of dementia, there are ways to soften its impact on patients and their families. Many families initially wish to keep a loved one with dementia at home, but they soon become overwhelmed by the problems this presents. Families can overcome many of these problems if they have a good understanding of dementia and know some effective strategies. Fortunately, materials and programs are available that can provide families with information about how to better manage the home care of patients with dementia. Studies have shown that families that learn about dementia and effective management and coping strategies are able to delay placing their loved one in a nursing home almost a year longer than those without similar knowledge and resources.

Many families that are determined to keep their loved one at home become overwhelmed because they fail to use the services of the various agencies and organizations in the community that offer assistance to patients with dementia and their families. Respite care and adult day care programs can provide caregivers with much-needed relief from the seemingly constant demands of monitoring and caring for a cognitively impaired person. Unfortunately, families are often unaware of these services.

Support groups are an important part of the care of patients with dementia and their families. Many of the emotional conflicts and burdens associated with the constant care of a loved one with dementia can be eased by sharing feelings and information with others facing the same challenges.

People also need to become more aware of the encouraging developments in the area of prevention. They need to understand the relationship between dementia and modifiable risk factors such as hypertension.

SUGGESTIONS FOR CONGREGATIONAL PROGRAMS

- Sponsor a special program on dementia. A neurologist or other physician familiar with dementia can provide helpful information and should be able to respond to the various questions and concerns of the audience. You may wish to provide free blood pressure checks before or after the physician's talk. This will help people make the connection between hypertension and dementia.
- Sponsor a special program on the community resources available to patients and families affected by dementia. This could include information about the various living arrangements appropriate for dementia patients at different stages of their condition. A social worker or case manager from a hospital, nursing home, or home health agency could serve as your featured speaker.
- Compile and distribute a list of agencies and organizations in your community that provide services appropriate for patients and families affected by dementia. This could include support groups, respite care programs, adult day care centers, and home health agencies.
- Compile and distribute a list of books and materials that offer families advice on managing dementia. One book that should be on this list is *The 36-Hour Day*, by Nancy L. Mace and Peter V. Rabins (see the suggested readings for more information).
- Sponsor a weekly or monthly "Caregivers' Night Out" program. Families that are caring for a loved one suffering from dementia get few opportunities to meet their own social needs. Even if they are using adult day care, the family usually have to spend their evenings caring for and monitoring their cognitively impaired relative. Most would welcome the opportunity to have an evening to go out if they knew that their afflicted relative was receiving good care arranged by their congregation.

EXAMPLES OF CONGREGATIONAL PROGRAMS

The lay health educator for a Catholic congregation organized a Saturday morning program on dementia. She invited Dr. M., a neurologist known for his work with Alzheimer disease and other dementias, to be the featured speaker. Free blood pressure checks and low-fat snacks were provided.

Dr. M. began his presentation with information about many of the discouraging aspects of dementia. He did not paint a very pretty picture of dementia because he felt that people needed to have an accurate understanding of the challenges facing dementia patients and their families. Dr. M. then moved on to some of the treatments and resources that can improve the lives of dementia patients and their families. He did not hold out the promise of a cure, but he did explain how some of the problems could be minimized by learning certain strategies and techniques. During the discussion following Dr. M.'s presentation, many important questions were asked. Another interesting development during this part of the program was an informal exchange of information among participants about various resources and strategies that they had found to be helpful in dealing with dementia. Although this discussion had not been planned, it proved to be valuable to many of the people in attendance.

Another valuable congregational program on dementia was coordinated by lay health educators representing four churches (Christian and Missionary Alliance, Episcopal, Lutheran, and Presbyterian). The representatives organized an afternoon program on short- and long-term care options for patients who have dementia or are physically frail. They put together a panel of experts that included a physician who specialized in geriatrics, a discharge planner from the local hospital, the director of an adult day care center, and an administrator from an agency that provided in-home medical and personal care services. The pastor of the Presbyterian church hosting the program served as the moderator.

The physician began the program and touched on many important aspects of medical care for cognitively impaired and physically frail persons. He also explained how factors other than the underlying illness must be considered when searching for long-term care options. For example, the functional abilities (ability to care for oneself) and the availability of a care-giver in the home must be considered.

The discharge planner then discussed the options she has when help-ing the patient and family identify the appropriate setting. Among these were the patient's home with home health care provided by professionals, an assisted living facility, and a skilled nursing facility. She provided the audience with information on the costs of the different options and the cri-teria used to determine insurance or Medicare payment for the services.

Next, the director of the adult day care center described the services provided in that type of setting. She also handed out and reviewed a list of the terms frequently used by professionals discussing care options for the chronically ill patient. Finally, the administrator of the home health agency shared information on the medical and personal care services his organi-zation could provide.

The pastor served as moderator for the question-and-answer part of the program. The questions from the audience revealed that there was great interest in the topic and that many people were unaware of the resources in their community. It was clear that the lay health educators had provided a valuable service by bringing together a group of professionals whose expertise spanned virtually the entire range of issues on the topic of caring for cognitively impaired and physically frail elderly persons.

INFORMATION RESOURCES

Many communities have a chapter of the Alzheimer's Association. You can call the national office of the Alzheimer's Association (1-800-272-3900) to find the location of the nearest chapter. This organization can provide a wide variety of materials and information about other community re-sources. These are some of the materials you will find at most Alzheimer's Association offices:

- Brochures listing the warning signs of Alzheimer disease and related dementias
- Brochures describing the steps to take to determine whether a per-son has Alzheimer disease

- Brochures providing an overview of Alzheimer disease and related dementias
- Brochures describing how family members can respond to persons with Alzheimer disease
- Brochures providing advice on how to plan for the future of a person with Alzheimer disease

The Alzheimer's Association can also provide information about other resources, including the following:

- Telephone helplines
- Guest speakers for congregational and community programs
- Professionals with expertise in dementia
- Support services for families caring for an Alzheimer patient in their home
- Support groups for patients and families
- Living arrangement options for patients with Alzheimer disease

Another source of information and materials about Alzheimer disease is the Alzheimer's Disease Education and Referral Center, a service of the National Institute on Aging, which can be called at 1-800-438-4380. In addition, information on dementia and the resources available for caregivers can be found in *The 36-Hour Day*, by Nancy L. Mace and Peter V. Rabins (see the suggested readings).

The following Internet Web sites provide information on dementia: < http://www.alz.org/ > and < http://www.alzheimers.org/ > .

10

Advance Directives

Every adult has the moral and legal right to accept or refuse recommended medical treatments. Each person can decide what to accept and what to reject. Physicians, hospitals, and nursing homes must respect the wishes of competent adults, even if they disagree with certain decisions. Some people may decide that they do not want to accept a medical treatment or be on a type of life support system if they are terminally ill or have a progressive illness and functional or cognitive disabilities.

Although patients always have the right to make decisions about medical care, it is possible that an injury or illness will prevent them from making a decision or communicating their wishes. Often the hardest decisions about life-sustaining or invasive treatments must be made by family members who have never asked their loved ones what treatment they would or would not want. Therefore, it is advisable for adults of all ages to do some advance planning and use one or more advance directives to convey their wishes and decisions. The two most important ones are the living will and the durable power of attorney for health care/surrogate decision maker.

A *living will* is a document that allows you to specify which treatments you would or would not want should you become incapacitated *and* be terminally ill or in a persistent vegetative state without probable recovery. In most U.S. states, a living will applies only in these very restricted situations. For example, you might not wish to be put on a ventilator, have a feeding tube inserted, or be given aggressive antibiotic therapy should you be terminally ill or in a persistent vegetative state.

It is extremely difficult to anticipate all the medical conditions you might encounter or all the treatments that might be available. Therefore, it is advisable to have a *durable power of attorney for health care* (sometimes called a *health care surrogate* or *surrogate decision maker*) in addition to a living will. This document allows you to appoint a family member or a friend to act as your agent and make decisions about your medical care should you become incapacitated. It does not require that you be terminally ill or in a persistent vegetative state, only that you be incapacitated and unable to make or communicate your own decisions. Therefore, it is more broadly applicable than a living will. The person appointed by you is legally obligated to see that *your* wishes are followed. Your appointed agent is legally obligated to choose not what he or she thinks is best, but what you would choose, if you could make the decision.

On admission, hospitals and nursing homes must provide patients with information about advance directives and give them an opportunity to complete these documents. However, usually this is not the best time to consider such matters carefully and make important decisions. It is difficult for patients to gather all the information about the various medical circumstances they may encounter, carefully weigh their options, and then communicate their wishes to their family and physician at the time of admission. These matters should be investigated and the documents completed at a time when a person is not seriously ill or requires admission to a hospital or nursing home. Later, the documents can be revised as needed.

"Do not resuscitate" orders can also be a part of advance medical planning. These orders, placed on the hospital chart, inform the hospital staff that the patient does not wish to undergo cardiopulmonary resuscitation should he or she experience cardiac arrest. Patients' physicians can provide them with additional information and advice about this subject.

THE RISKS OF FAILING TO USE ADVANCE DIRECTIVES

People who fail to use advance directives run the risk of receiving treatment or medical care that they do not want. Without the appropriate directives, they could be kept alive under conditions they would find completely unacceptable, and major decisions about their medical care could be made by individuals who have entirely different values and expectations.

The absence of advance planning can also result in painful and destructive conflicts among family members. One member of a patient's family may feel strongly that the patient would not want to be kept on life support systems, whereas another family member may feel equally strongly that it would be wrong to withdraw the support. If the patient has not completed a living will or appointed someone to make these decisions, the hospital and doctor must choose a decision maker from a predetermined list, who may not make decisions reflecting the patient's wishes.

WHAT CAN BE DONE TO PREVENT LOSS OF CONTROL OVER MEDICAL DECISIONS?

Most people are aware of advance directives—at least the living will—and are in favor of using them. However, surveys show that only a small proportion of adults has formally expressed their wishes and had the appropriate forms completed and witnessed. One reason for people failing to complete the forms is that both physicians and patients are reluctant to broach the subject; each would prefer that the other raise the issue. Therefore, it is important to encourage people to discuss this matter with their physician. They should not wait for their physician to take the initiative.

Some people mistakenly believe that they must have an attorney to prepare a living will or a durable power of attorney for health care and are reluctant to incur the costs associated with hiring one. Fortunately, advance directives do not require the services of an attorney. Forms can be obtained from hospitals, home health agencies, and several national organizations. Furthermore, the forms obtained from these organizations can be modified to suit the wishes of each person. Another option is for people to write out their own advance directives. These are legal and acceptable directives as long as they are properly witnessed by two adults, only one of whom may be a member of the immediate family and neither of whom may be designated as the surrogate decision maker.

Another misconception held by some people is that they will permanently lose control of decisions about their medical care once a living will or durable power of attorney for health care has been prepared and signed. They think they are signing a document that is permanent and irrevocable. It is important to inform people that these documents are utilized only when patients are unable to communicate their wishes. Furthermore, people need to understand that they can change or revoke an advance directive at any time.

People also need to be encouraged to discuss their wishes and feelings about end-of-life matters with family members or other designated decision makers. These individuals need to know that the documents exist and that they were executed after careful consideration of the medical circumstances and options. A statement or declaration of personal values completed by the patient can be helpful to family members who need to understand the patient's wishes and decisions. Additionally, a statement of values can serve as a helpful guide for a person who has the durable power of attorney for health care.

SUGGESTIONS FOR CONGREGATIONAL PROGRAMS

- Use congregational bulletins and mailings to provide members of your congregation with information about advance directives. Information and sample forms can be obtained from hospitals and home health agencies.
- Sponsor a program on advance directives. A physician or nurse can provide information about the medical circumstances patients might encounter and the decisions they might face. A hospital social worker can also offer advice on this topic.
- Arrange for an attorney to meet individually or collectively with members of your congregation to offer advice on how to personalize these documents.
- Sponsor a program on ethical decision making. This could be led by the clergy and include examples of statements/declarations of values.
- Arrange for members of your congregation to videotape their wishes and instructions on end-of-life matters. This videotape could then be used to supplement written documents if the situation arises.

EXAMPLES OF CONGREGATIONAL PROGRAMS

Lay health educators from three churches (Baptist, Methodist, and Presbyterian) worked together to sponsor a program on advance directives for members of their congregations and others in the community who were interested in the topic. The meeting was held on a Tuesday morning in the fellowship hall of the Presbyterian church. An attorney who specialized in elder law and a social worker who was director of social services at the local hospital volunteered to speak at this program. More than sixty people gathered for the meeting. Following introductions by the lay health educators, the speakers discussed the basic aspects of advance directives. They provided examples of medical situations people might encounter and the options they would have in these situations. The speakers then invited members of the audience to ask questions. Following the group question-and-answer period, refreshments were served, and the attorney and social worker made themselves available on a one-to-one basis for those who had additional questions.

During a Shabbat service, the rabbi asked the members attending the synagogue to stay for a few minutes after the service to hear brief presentations by a physician (who was not a member of the congregation) and an attorney (who was a member). The doctor, an oncologist, offered several examples of situations in which patients with terminal illnesses who had lost their ability to communicate with others were forced to receive medical treatment that they probably did not want. However, because they had not prepared advance directives expressing their wishes, the doctor and hospital were forced to continue the treatment. He strongly implored members of the congregation to avoid these situations by completing a living will and designating a trusted individual as their surrogate decision maker. The attorney provided additional information about these documents and further encouraged members to use them. The rabbi reinforced their advice by also recommending that members take these measures to ensure that their wishes about end-of-life matters will be enforced.

INFORMATION RESOURCES

Hospitals and home health agencies can provide copies of advance directives, and many will arrange for knowledgeable speakers to give presentations to community groups. Many attorneys will also volunteer their time to speak to groups about advance directives.

Choice In Dying, a national not-for-profit organization, can also provide information about advance directives. This organization offers state-specific advance directive packages for a small fee. These materials are designed to conform to the laws of the specified state. Choice In Dying can be contacted at 1-800-989-WILL (9455). Another resource is the American Association of Retired Persons (AARP). AARP publishes a booklet entitled "Shape Your Health Care Future with Health Care Advance Directives." AARP can be contacted at 1-800-424-3410.

The following Internet Web site has information on advance directives: < http://www.choices.org/ > .

11

Accidents and Falls

Accidents and falls are frequently overlooked as major health problems associated with aging. However, both the incidence and severity of falls increase with age, and accidents are among the ten leading causes of death among older adults. Almost one-third of adults aged 65 and over who are living at home will experience a fall each year, and approximately one in forty of these falls will result in hospitalization.

Many different factors can contribute to the increased susceptibility to experiencing a fall in older adults. Some of these are associated with the aging process, including changes in postural control and gait. Also, some of the medical disorders that occur more frequently in old age can contribute to falls. For example, the muscle weakness and sensory deficits from a stroke can lead to instability. Medications can also contribute to falls. However, many falls are the result of environmental factors and could be prevented by making changes in the living environment.

THE DANGERS OF IGNORING INFORMATION
ON ACCIDENTS AND FALLS

There are many complications of falls, including fractures and neurological injuries. Additionally, falls and their complications frequently result in serious functional limitations. People who have fallen and suffered injuries may experience permanently impaired mobility. In addition, the fear of falling, which often follows a fall, may result in curtailment of activities, leading to muscle weakening and, paradoxically, possibly further increasing the risk of future falls. People who fall are likely to experience a loss of independence and are at greater risk of being institutionalized.

WHAT CAN BE DONE TO REDUCE THE RISK OF ACCIDENTS AND FALLS?

Fortunately, patients, their families, and caregivers can make any number of changes in the living environments of older adults to reduce the risk of accidents and falls, such as the following:

- Remove throw rugs.
- Tack down large rugs and carpeting completely.
- Remove low furniture.
- Keep objects off the floor.
- Use nonslip polish on floors.
- Install handrails along both sides of stairs.
- Provide good illumination, especially on steps and landings.
- Make light switches easily accessible near doors and room entrances.
- Use nightlights in bedrooms, bathrooms, and hallways.
- Use nonskid rubber mats in showers or baths.
- Install handrails for baths and toilets.
- Keep water off the floors.
- Use bath or shower seats.
- Install raised toilet seats.
- Keep food and other necessary items on low, easy-to-reach shelves.

People can also reduce the risk of accidents and falls by using appropriate assistive devices (e.g., canes, walkers). Unfortunately, many people who would benefit from such devices fail to use them or do not use the most appropriate and effective ones.

SUGGESTIONS FOR CONGREGATIONAL PROGRAMS

- Sponsor a program on home safety, mobility, and assistive devices. A physical therapist could be one of your featured speakers, along with a representative from a company that provides in-home medical supplies and equipment.

- Recruit and train a group of volunteers who would be willing to conduct home safety checks for members of the congregation. Social workers from the local hospital or a home health agency can assist in their training.

- Recruit and train a group of volunteers who are willing to use their knowledge and skills to make minor modifications to improve home safety (e.g., install grab bars and handrails).

- Organize a group of volunteers who are willing to provide basic house and yard maintenance for people who are physically incapacitated. This could be done on a short- or long-term basis, depending on the congregation's needs and resources. This service could help some individuals avoid or delay placement in a nursing home or other long-term care facility.

- Use congregational bulletins and mailings to provide members with helpful suggestions and reminders about home safety. Home health agencies and companies that provide in-home medical supplies may have materials that you can distribute.

EXAMPLES OF CONGREGATIONAL PROGRAMS

A congregational program designed to reduce accidents and injuries was coordinated by two lay health educators for a Baptist church with many elderly members. They inserted in the church's bulletin and its newsletter, which is mailed to all members of the church, a list of suggestions on how to reduce the risk of accidents in the home. Accompanying this list was an announcement of a special program on the same topic that would be given during the next regularly scheduled meeting of the church's seniors group. They also invited members of nearby churches and a retirement center to attend the program. A gerontologist from the local college was the featured speaker, and a physical therapist from the local hospital was available to answer questions. Additionally, the lay health educators and a few other members of the church offered to conduct home safety checks and modifications for older adults who needed assistance.

The lay health educator at a Presbyterian church worked with members of an adult Sunday school class to initiate a program on how to prevent falls and accidents. The lay health educator arranged for a representative from a home health agency to speak to the class about strategies for reducing the risk of accidents and falls in the home. She also distributed materials that could be used to evaluate home safety. Class members felt it was important to share this information with others in the church and arranged for it to be included in the church bulletin and monthly newsletter. They also decided to reach out to residents of the retirement complex next to the church. With the help of the home health agency representative, the class organized a special program on home safety. They distributed informational materials, and several members of the church volunteered to help residents who wanted assistance in evaluating their apartments or making minor modifications.

INFORMATION RESOURCES

The best resources for programs on home safety can be found in local institutions and agencies. Hospitals and home health agencies can provide materials for your programs and help you find professionals who can serve as guest speakers.

12

Influenza and Pneumonia

Influenza, usually called the flu, is a viral infection of the respiratory tract. Symptoms generally include fever, chills, dry cough, and muscle aches. For most of the 35 to 50 million Americans it strikes each year, influenza is not a serious illness. Although certainly unpleasant, most people are ill for only a few days and return to their regular level of activity within a couple of weeks. However, influenza is a serious health problem for high-risk groups, especially the elderly. In a typical year, 150,000 Americans are hospitalized due to influenza, and as many as 20,000 die of influenza and its complications. (Some years the figure has exceeded 40,000, and in 1918–19 more than half a million Americans died of influenza and its complications.)

Pneumonia is an infection of one or both lungs. It is most commonly caused by bacteria and, more rarely, by viruses, fungi, and other microorganisms. *Pneumococcal pneumonia*, a bacterial infection, is one of the most common types of pneumonia. Symptoms include fever, cough producing sputum, chest pain when inhaling, shortness of breath, headache, weakness, and fatigue. Although hospitalizations and deaths due to pneumonia have decreased dramatically since the advent of antibiotics, pneumonia still results in approximately half a million hospitalizations each year and is one of the ten leading causes of death.

THE RISKS OF IGNORING INFORMATION ON INFLUENZA AND PNEUMONIA

The greatest danger of ignoring information on influenza and pneumonia is that people in high-risk groups, especially elderly persons, will not recognize these illnesses as being serious and potentially fatal and thus will fail to take proper preventive steps. For both influenza and pneumonia, the most effective method of prevention is vaccination. Most hospitalizations and deaths resulting from influenza and pneumonia could be prevented by vaccinations. People should get influenza vaccinations on an annual basis. Vaccinations for pneumonia provide long-term protection and may be needed no more often than once every five to ten years. (Recommendations vary. People should check with their physician for more specific guidelines.)

In spite of the demonstrated effectiveness of influenza vaccinations and the fact that Medicare provides reimbursement, less than half of all Medicare beneficiaries get these vaccinations. The percentage is even less among African-American beneficiaries, with only about 25 percent obtaining vaccinations.

The failure of people in high-risk groups to receive the recommended vaccination is costly in both human and economic terms. Thousands of lives and billions of dollars could be saved every year if more people would get these vaccinations.

WHAT CAN BE DONE TO PREVENT INFLUENZA AND PNEUMONIA?

It does not appear that economic barriers are responsible for the low number of people receiving vaccinations. Vaccinations are inexpensive, reimbursed by Medicare, and relatively easy to obtain. Instead, the major barriers seem to be erroneous beliefs, such as the following:

- Influenza is not a serious illness.
- Pneumonia can always be successfully treated with antibiotics.
- People can get influenza from an influenza vaccination.
- An influenza vaccination is effective for several years.

These beliefs interfere with people taking the necessary steps to avoid what can be serious, life-threatening illnesses. People in high-risk groups need to be given information that will encourage them to get vaccinations for influenza and pneumonia. These are the high-risk groups that need this information:

- People 65 years of age or older
- People of any age who have chronic medical conditions, including diabetes; heart, lung, or kidney disease; or weakened immune systems
- People of any age who live or work with members of high-risk groups and thus could easily transmit influenza

SUGGESTIONS FOR CONGREGATIONAL PROGRAMS

- Make a special effort to distribute information to classes and groups that consist primarily of older adults.
- Provide members of your congregation and community with information about the times and places they can receive vaccinations. This information can be obtained from your public health department or local hospitals.
- Arrange to offer influenza vaccinations at your congregational facility. The public health department, local hospital, or a home health agency should be able to provide nurses and supplies.
- Arrange transportation to sites that provide vaccinations if you are unable to arrange for vaccinations to be given on-site.
- Coordinate your congregational efforts with national public awareness campaigns. The national campaign to educate people about the benefits of influenza vaccinations usually starts in mid-October.
- Use congregational bulletins and mailings to give members information about the potentially serious consequences of influenza and pneumonia and the definite benefits of vaccinations.

EXAMPLES OF CONGREGATIONAL PROGRAMS

Two members of a Baptist church who had been through a lay health educator training program coordinated an influenza vaccination program for their congregation. Their first goal was to inform the congregation of the dangers of influenza and the protection an annual vaccination would provide. To achieve this goal, the lay health educators placed information about the dangers of influenza in congregational bulletins and mailings. They also made a special effort to target older adults by making announcements and distributing additional materials to the church's seniors group. Next, they arranged for nurses from a health care agency to come to the church and offer vaccinations. They publicized this program by distributing to their congregation's members small packages of tissues that had stickers with the slogan "Get the Facts, Stop Flu in Its Tracks" attached to them. In addition, in Sunday school classes, they showed a ten-minute videotape in which a local physician spoke of the dangers of influenza and strongly encouraged people to get their vaccinations. More than fifty adults got vaccinated at the church, and many others reported that the information they had received had prompted them to request vaccinations from their physicians.

A volunteer from a Catholic church felt that the members of a largely Hispanic mission sponsored by her church were likely to be unaware of the dangers of influenza and that it would be wise to offer vaccinations to all age groups in this congregation. Working closely with the public health department, she arranged to have free vaccinations offered immediately after the Sunday service. The response was overwhelming. Ninety members were vaccinated, and many others wished to be vaccinated, but, unfortunately, the health department's staff had brought only ninety doses. However, pleased with the enthusiastic response of the congregation, the staff offered to return the following Sunday to provide additional vaccinations. Another ninety members were vaccinated at that time.

INFORMATION RESOURCES

Hospitals, home health agencies, and public health departments are good local resources for programs on influenza and pneumonia. In many communities, these organizations will sponsor annual influenza vaccination campaigns and welcome the participation of religious congregations. The Centers for Disease Control is a good national resource that can provide much of the information you will need for your programs. The telephone number for its fax information service is 1-888-CDC-FAXX (232-3299).

The American Lung Association also can provide information on influenza and pneumonia. The association can be reached at 1-800-LUNG-USA (800-586-4872).

The following Internet Web sites provide information on influenza and pneumonia: <http://www.lungusa.org/> and <http://www.medicare.gov/fightflu/fightflu.html>.

13

Medication Management

Noncompliance with prescribed treatment regimens, especially medications, is one of the most persistent and vexing problems physicians and other health professionals encounter. Studies have shown that as many as 50 percent of patients fail to take their medications as prescribed. The problem is even greater for older adults, in large part because they are likely to have multiple chronic diseases and thus multiple medications.

Numerous factors contribute to the high incidence of noncompliance, and many can be traced to communication problems between patients and their physicians. Often patients do not understand why their doctor has prescribed a certain medication. They may not understand what it is being used for and its benefits. They also may not be aware of the risks of not taking the medication. Unpleasant side effects also may lead to noncompliance. Frequently patients who experience unpleasant side effects stop taking their medication without informing their physician.

Noncompliance also increases as the number of medications prescribed increases. Because elderly persons take an average of five to seven medications, it is not surprising that many have difficulty organizing and taking all of their medications exactly as prescribed.

Finally, noncompliance can be related to economic status. Some medications are quite expensive, and individuals with limited financial resources may be forced to choose between buying a prescribed medicine and purchasing another needed product or service.

THE RISKS OF IGNORING INFORMATION
ON MEDICATION MANAGEMENT

The most serious danger of failing to take a medication as instructed is that the disorder or condition for which it is prescribed will not be controlled and thus the patient will be at risk of developing more serious medical problems. For example, patients with hypertension who fail to take their antihypertensive medication on a regular basis are increasing their chances of suffering a stroke or heart attack. Another danger is that if some medications are taken improperly, patients may develop new medical problems, such as mental confusion or injuries suffered from a fall because of an imbalance related to adverse effects on brain function.

WHAT CAN BE DONE TO PREVENT PROBLEMS
WITH MEDICATION MANAGEMENT?

Medications generally can be managed effectively if patients follow these recommendations:

- Understand why their physician has prescribed a medication. If patients do not understand, they should ask. They should know what the medication is for, how to take it, and what to expect.
- Write down the information and instructions provided by their physician. Patients should take notes about the prescribed medication while they are in the doctor's office. (The form in Appendix F can be used to assist in this regard.)
- Ask about foods and drinks that should be avoided while taking the medication(s).
- Ask their primary care physician to review all of their medications. Patients should take their medications, or at least a list of all their medications, to office visits. Over-the-counter (nonprescription) drugs should also be included.
- Report any unexpected or unpleasant side effects to their doctor.
- Use one pharmacist or pharmacy for all of their medications and accept medication counseling when it is offered by a pharmacist. If

patients still have any questions about the medication, they should ask their pharmacist or physician.

- Ask their pharmacist to contact their doctor if they feel they cannot afford the medication that has been prescribed. The pharmacist and physician may be able to find a less expensive alternative.
- Take a relative or friend with them if they have difficulty talking with their physician or pharmacist.
- Use medication organizers or pill boxes if they have trouble remembering their medicine. These boxes can be purchased at pharmacies, or patients can construct their own.
- Keep a record of their medications. This should include information about the drug, what it is for, its color and shape, directions and cautions, and the times at which it should be taken. Appendix F provides a sample medication record.

SUGGESTIONS FOR CONGREGATIONAL PROGRAMS

- Sponsor a program or series of programs on medication management with a local pharmacist who is a good communicator as your featured speaker. Among the topics that could be covered in a series on medications are communicating with your pharmacist and physician about medications; commonly prescribed drugs and common mistakes people make when taking these medications; and nonprescription medications.
- Schedule a meeting about medications. Encourage members of your congregation to put all their medications, including nonprescription ones, in a bag and bring them to the meeting. Have a pharmacist available to review and discuss the various medications.
- Provide members of your congregation with medication record forms. These are easy and simple to design or copy. Appendix F provides a sample form.
- Offer members of your congregation medication organizers. The organizers can be purchased at pharmacies or constructed by volunteers. Some hospitals and pharmaceutical companies may be willing to donate a small number of the organizers.
- Use congregational bulletins and mailings to remind members of

your congregation of the need to take their medications as directed. Information on some of the more commonly prescribed medications, which can be obtained from the local hospital or pharmacies, can be included.

EXAMPLES OF CONGREGATIONAL PROGRAMS

An informative program on medication management was coordinated by volunteers from four churches. They sponsored a Saturday morning program on several health topics, including medications. In spite of rain and severe weather warnings, more than forty people attended. The first part of the program, held in the sanctuary of one of the churches, consisted of presentations by a panel of health care professionals. Panelists included a pharmacist, a physician, a dietitian, and a physical therapist. A volunteer from one of the churches served as the moderator for the panel. Members of the audience were encouraged to ask the panelists questions or write their questions on a card and have the moderator direct the questions to the appropriate panelist. Several questions on medications were asked, and it proved quite helpful to have not only a pharmacist but also a physician and a dietitian available to respond to different issues related to medications.

For the second part of the program, each professional was given a small room in the education wing of the church and members of the audience were invited to participate in small group or individual discussions with the professionals. Most of the audience stayed for this part and took advantage of the opportunity to talk with health care professionals in a setting that was more relaxed and less hurried than the typical office or pharmacy visit.

Another excellent educational program on medication management was held as part of a five-week health education series sponsored by a large Protestant church. Each Wednesday night during the month of January, members were invited to attend these sessions, which began immediately after the regularly scheduled church supper. Almost a hundred members attended the session on medications. This program was held in the chapel and featured a pharmacist from the local hospital as the guest speaker. The pharmacist received an enthusiastic introduction by the lay health educator. She first became acquainted with the pharmacist when he led the lay health educator training workshop on medication management, and she knew that the audience would find him to be as interesting and informative as she had.

The pharmacist emphasized several points during his presentation, but the overarching message was that people need to take responsibility for understanding their medications. He stated that people need to take the initiative in discussing their medications with their doctor and pharmacist and that they should not be shy about asking questions. He encouraged the members of the congregation to take their medications, or at least a complete list of their medications (including over-the-counter medications), to their visits with their doctor or to the pharmacy when getting a new prescription filled. In addition, he suggested that they keep a chart describing their medications, what they are for, and when they should be taken. (The lay health educator provided sample charts for those who were interested.) He also repeatedly emphasized that they should not hesitate to call their pharmacist whenever they had a question about their medications.

During the question-and-answer session that followed, the pharmacist was asked several questions about specific medications, including generic drugs. The audience seemed enthusiastic about his presentation and thanked both him and the lay health educator for offering the program.

INFORMATION RESOURCES

Multiple copies of the informative brochure "Prescription Medicines and You: A Consumer Guide" can be obtained from the National Council on Patient Information and Education (NCPIE): NCPIE Rx Guide, 666 Eleventh Street, N.W., Suite 810, Washington, DC 20001-4542, (202) 347-6711. In addition, local pharmacies can supply information sheets on various medications.

The following Internet Web sites provide information on medication management: <http://www.usp.org/> and <http://www.pharmacyandyou .org/>.

PATIENT ADVOCACY

14

Developing a Program
to Train Patient Advocates

Health education programs and medical screenings held in religious congregations and coordinated by lay leaders are certainly effective methods for helping people maintain their health, but there is a need for another type of health ministry involving laypersons. Within most congregations, a number of persons are ill and have difficulty managing various aspects of their health and medical care. Coping with chronic conditions and navigating through a complex health system can be quite challenging. It can be especially challenging for elderly persons and others who have multiple health conditions and thus require a variety of medications or treatments.

For many people, one way of handling these challenges is to have a family member or friend accompany them to their appointments and serve as an extra pair of eyes and ears. Some individuals are particularly fortunate in this regard because they have family members or friends with experience in the medical field who can accompany them to their appointments and provide ongoing support. However, too many people are forced to confront the challenges of managing their chronic conditions and medical care alone. These are the individuals who can benefit greatly from a volunteer who provides the same type of assistance and support a concerned family member, especially one who is familiar with medical matters, can offer.

Working closely with health care professionals and religious leaders, we developed a training program for members of religious congregations who were interested in serving as patient advocates or health care partners. As we prepared this program, we received valuable advice from physicians, nurses, social workers, clergy, and patients. They shared with us the strategies and resources that can be used by patients and those who want to assist them as they cope with their illnesses, and we have incorporated the best and most useful suggestions into our training materials.

THE GOALS OF PATIENT ADVOCACY

The goal of the patient advocate program is to train people to work on a one-to-one basis with older adults and others who need assistance managing chronic illnesses and medical conditions. The primary responsibility of patient advocates is to serve as an extra pair of eyes and ears when patients are interacting with their physicians, facilitating the flow of information between patients and physicians. This exchange of information is the key to effective treatment and management of chronic illnesses. For good, comprehensive medical care to be provided, it is essential that patients give their physicians and other health care providers complete, accurate reports of their symptoms and the treatment regimens they are following. Likewise, it is important for the physicians to provide patients with complete reports of their findings and recommendations in terms that can be easily understood and remembered.

Once medical information has been exchanged, patients often need assistance in following their physician's recommendations. For example, patients often find it difficult to remember follow-up appointments or consistently comply with their doctor's recommendations about medications. Patient advocates can help patients organize their schedules and medicines and then provide further assistance by telephone or brief visits. Additionally, they can discuss with patients steps to prevent additional medical problems (e.g., injuries resulting from falls) and how to maintain control over decisions about their medical care should they become incapacitated (e.g., use of advance directives). Patient advocates can even provide emotional support and reassurance for patients. However, patient advocates are not expected to provide any financial support, nor are they to reap any financial benefits from their work.

THE SPECIAL QUALITIES OF A PATIENT ADVOCATE

Although the time demands on patient advocates do not have to be great and the training required to serve as a patient advocate is not extensive, several special qualities are necessary to serve in this capacity. First, patient advocates must be willing to listen to and talk about difficult issues. Some of the things they hear about and discuss with patients and physicians may not be pleasant, yet these matters must be dealt with openly and professionally in order to facilitate the best possible care for the patient. Furthermore, patient advocates often are entrusted with sensitive information that must be treated with *absolute confidentiality*. This point cannot be emphasized enough. Patient advocates must understand and accept this responsibility. The information they hear cannot be shared with anyone other than the patient unless they are clearly instructed to do so.

Second, patient advocates must be able to earn the trust of both patients and medical professionals. Although we can provide individuals with the knowledge and skills to serve as patient advocates, their effectiveness will be greatly limited if they do not have the trust and respect of patients and health care providers.

Third, patient advocates must be able to respect not only the privacy of patients but also their wishes. Patient advocates may encounter situations in which the wishes or values of the patient conflict with their own. In these situations, patient advocates must be willing to set aside their own feelings and act on behalf of the patient. It is the patient advocate's responsibility to act as the agent or representative of the patient.

It is also important that patient advocates not bring their own personal agendas regarding medicine into their work. The role of the patient advocate is to serve as a facilitator, not as an adversary of physicians, nurses, or hospitals. Although patient advocates may need to be assertive and persistent in some of their efforts, they still need to feel comfortable about working within the health care system.

THE PERSONAL SIDE OF THE PATIENT ADVOCATE PROGRAM

One summer I (WDH) spent a month going on hospital rounds with the medical team of an experienced physician who also serves as an instructor in a family practice residency program. Accompanying him on the rounds were two young physicians. I found all three of these physicians to be excellent communicators who took ample time with their patients. They encouraged their patients to share all their concerns and ask questions. In turn, they tried to respond to all the questions and concerns they heard with clear answers and easy-to-understand recommendations. Nevertheless, in spite of the physicians' best efforts, many of their patients were reluctant to disclose all their concerns and ask questions when they did not understand something. Invisible barriers were blocking the flow of information necessary for good medical care.

What I had witnessed in the hospital was frustrating to all who were involved. On many occasions, the physicians and I knew that the patients had not disclosed all the information that was needed to provide them with the best and most appropriate care. We knew that there were personal, family, or financial factors that would interfere with the patients' recommended treatment, but we were not told enough about these factors. Frequently it appeared that patients did not understand what the physicians had told them about their diagnosis and treatment options, yet they would not voice their confusion or uncertainty.

I was certain that many patients felt more frustrated than the physicians. Patients who were confused and wanted more information about their illness did not know what questions to ask. Perhaps they did not feel they had enough information to ask the appropriate questions, or they were too anxious to think clearly about the situation. Additionally, some patients thought that the physicians would not understand or care about personal factors that would prevent them from following the recommendations they had received. These patients form part of that very large group of patients who fail to benefit fully from medical treatment because they do not or cannot follow the advice of their physicians. Much of the time and effort that had gone into their treatment would yield virtually no benefits because of the problems resulting from poor communication.

When I discussed these experiences with Dr. Bennett, during one of

his visits to Florida when we were developing the health education program, I learned that he and his colleagues had experienced similar frus-
trations. Often their patients would not share important information with
them or would not ask questions when they were unclear about the treatments being recommended. Dr. Bennett said that with some patients, the
only time he could be relatively confident that he had all the information
he needed and that the patient understood and would follow his recommendations was when a concerned relative was present and actively involved. These concerned relatives often had helped the patients prepare a
list of questions and would assist them in articulating their concerns. They
also would write down information given to the patients about medications
and subsequent appointments.

Through further discussions with other physicians, I realized that this
was exactly the role I had played for my mother. On several occasions I was
with her when she met with the doctor. I helped her get organized for her
appointments so that she could cover all the subjects that needed to be discussed. We often made lists to be certain that we would not forget an important item. Sometimes during her meetings, she would be reluctant to express her concerns because her doctor appeared to be extremely busy and
she felt she should not take up too much of his time. When this occurred,
I would have to encourage her to speak up. When her doctor made recommendations, I would write down the information and make sure that
she and I had correctly understood what had been said. And following my
mother's doctor's appointments or discharges from the hospital, I would
visit or call to help remind her about her medications or next appointment.

From these experiences and conversations, we developed a training
program for volunteers from religious congregations who wanted to serve
as patient advocates or health partners. We were convinced then, and are
even more convinced today, that a patient advocate program can improve
the medical treatment and care of individuals with chronic illnesses. Furthermore, we now know that in most communities there are physicians,
nurses, pharmacists, and social workers who will assist in providing training for interested individuals.

Sponsoring a patient advocate program is potentially one of the most
valuable health services a congregation can offer its community. Every congregation has elderly or infirm individuals who do not have a spouse or
other family member to serve as their advocate. And many of the people

who do serve as advocates for family members do not know enough about medical treatments and health care services to be as effective as they would like to be. A patient advocate program, drawing on the resources of the congregation and local health care providers, can help people overcome many of the obstacles that can interfere with good medical care, and an active patient advocate program can serve as a reminder of the congregation's mission as a caring institution.

15

Establishing Productive
Partnerships with Patients

It is important for patient advocates to establish productive partnerships with the individuals they will be assisting. They need to develop good relationships in which the patients not only trust them and have confidence in their ability to help with medical matters but also feel comfortable sharing personal information with them.

DEVELOPING GOOD WORKING RELATIONSHIPS

Patient advocates need to establish good working relationships with the patients they are assisting. This is usually a two-step process: The first step is developing rapport with the patient; the second step is clarifying your role as a patient advocate.

Developing Rapport

As a patient advocate, the best way to begin a relationship with a patient is to say a few things about yourself (e.g., your previous work experience or some of your current activities) and why you wish to serve as a patient advocate (e.g., you have helped a relative or friend with their medical matters and found it rewarding). Although you should disclose enough information about yourself so that the patient feels comfortable with you, do not get too detailed. You should keep the focus on the patient and his or her needs. As you talk with the patient, try to create a relaxed atmosphere. Let the patient see that you are comfortable talking about health matters and related personal concerns.

Clarifying Your Role

As you begin to develop rapport with the person you will be assisting, suggest that it would be helpful for you to explain specifically what you will be capable of doing as a patient advocate. Let the patient know how you envision your role.

One of the first matters you need to address is the issue of confidentiality. Many people we talked to about the patient advocate program expressed the concern that some of their medical problems might be discussed with acquaintances in their congregation or community. Even though a patient advocate might have good intentions about sharing information (e.g., encouraging others to provide assistance), such disclosures can undermine, and even destroy, the relationship between the patient and the patient advocate. Therefore, it is imperative that you treat all information as absolutely confidential. Only if the patient clearly gives you permission to share personal and medical information should you do so. You should take the initiative in discussing this issue because some patients may be reluctant to say anything about it even if they have concerns.

It also is important for you to clarify your limitations. You should be certain that the patient realizes you are not a medical expert. You should not be expected to be the direct source of information about medical matters. Instead, your role is to help the patient obtain the necessary information from physicians and other appropriate sources.

In addition, you need to clarify financial matters. It is not the role of the patient advocate to provide financial support for the patient. If the patient has financial problems that interfere with his or her ability to obtain recommended treatment, you may help him or her bring this to the attention of the physician, hospital social worker, or an appropriate social service agency, but you should not be expected to provide or find sources of money yourself.

Another financial matter that needs to be addressed is the issue of a patient advocate receiving money or gifts for his or her efforts. This may be an unspoken concern of the patient's family members who are not close enough to monitor your activities. They may fear that you will obtain control over the patient's bank account and misuse the money. It is best to address this fear by suggesting that the patient send a letter to relatives. The sample letter in Exhibit 1 can serve as a guide. This letter should help the patient's family better understand your role and allay any fears about your involvement in finances.

EXHIBIT 1. Sample Letter to Family Members

Dear _____   Date: _____

I want to let you know about a new program I am participating in that should help me obtain better medical care. Although I am satisfied with the care I am receiving, I have realized that I could benefit from an extra pair of eyes and ears during appointments with my doctor. Sometimes I forget to mention some important things to my doctor, and sometimes I have difficulty remembering everything he or she tells me during the appointment. Recently I met with _____, a volunteer who has been trained to serve as a PATIENT ADVOCATE. He or she has offered to meet with me before my next doctor's appointment and then to accompany me to the appointment.

_____ and the other volunteers in this PATIENT ADVOCATE program come from my congregation and have been trained by doctors, nurses, and other health professionals at _____ (name of hospital).

Their primary responsibility is to help patients communicate more effectively with their physicians and help them follow through with the recommendations of the physicians (e.g., take medications on a regular schedule). They do not get involved in our financial matters, and they do not get paid for their assistance.

Sincerely,

GATHERING INFORMATION

After you feel you have established rapport with the patient and given him or her enough information about your background, your interest in the program, and what can be expected of you, you are ready to begin gathering information about the patient's medical concerns and any related matters. The following suggestions about interviewing may be helpful to you as you begin asking questions.

First of all, you need to let the patient see that you are carefully attending to what he or she is saying. Good attending behavior includes the following attributes:

- *Eye contact*: Show your interest and concern by keeping your eyes focused on the patient.
- *Attentive posture*: Show that you are interested in what the patient is saying by leaning forward slightly.
- *Repeating or rephrasing of key comments*: Demonstrate that you are listening carefully and that you understand what is being said by repeating or rephrasing key comments. This also enables you to correct any misunderstandings.

Start by asking open-ended questions (e.g., "How can I be of help to you?" or "What is your greatest concern about your health?"). The advantage of open-ended questions is that you may discover some concerns you had not anticipated and would not have learned about if you had asked only specific, closed-ended questions. Some individuals will have difficulty responding to general, open-ended questions. When this occurs, switch to more specific questions (e.g., "What has the doctor told you about your condition?" or "What medications or treatments has your doctor recommended?").

Do not hesitate to speak up if you are confused by something the patient has said. If you do not understand a term or are uncertain about what the patient means, tell him or her that you are confused. This will let the patient see that you are genuinely interested in understanding what he or she is saying.

If the patient expresses a sense of loss or emotional pain related to his or her illness, do not try to provide immediate relief or reassurance. Give the patient ample opportunity to talk about his or her fears or losses. The danger of offering reassurance too quickly is that the patient is likely to think that you do not, or even do not wish to, understand his or her feelings. Or the patient may think that you simply do not wish to hear about his or her unpleasant feelings.

Do not rush to fill silent periods in your conversations. Give the patient time to think and respond. These silent periods can be valuable to both of you. He or she may need time to reflect on some issues you have raised, and you can use these periods both to review what has been discussed thus far and to observe the patient's nonverbal behavior. If you think the patient's eyes or facial expression reveals a certain emotion, share your observations. For example, if you think you detect fear, gently ask if this is what he or she is experiencing.

Finally, try not to be surprised or shocked by the unexpected. You may assume that the patient should feel a certain way because that is how you would feel or because you know how other people have reacted under circumstances similar to the patient's. Although it is helpful to draw on your own experiences or those of others, it is important to recognize that not everyone reacts in the same manner.

16

Preparing to Meet with the Physician

Many patients have had the experience of coming out of a meeting with their physician feeling more confused than when they went in. It is not unusual for patients to report that they do not completely understand their illness or what they should do to manage their condition more effectively, even though they have had several meetings with their doctor. Many factors can contribute to this confusion and uncertainty. These are some of the obstacles or problems frequently mentioned by patients:

- *Medical terminology*: "My doctor acted like I should understand the terminology he was using. I would have felt stupid telling him I didn't."
- *Doctor's schedule*: "The doctor seemed too busy to discuss all of my concerns. He looked rushed, and there were so many other patients in his waiting room."
- *Patient's anxiety*: "I was so nervous about my situation that I forgot to tell him some important things."
- *Patient's attitude*: "I find it difficult to question or be assertive with my doctor. It's easier to just listen quietly."
- *Doctor's interview style*: "My doctor's questions led me away from some of the things I had intended to discuss with him."
- *Information overload*: "There was just too much information. I was overwhelmed."
- *Problems with memory*: "I understood what he said, but by the time I got home I had forgotten most of it."

These and other problems can interfere with effective communication between a patient and his or her doctor. But there are ways to avoid most of these problems. By taking the time to prepare for an appointment, organizing the information that needs to be discussed, being assertive during the appointment, and carefully recording the information given by the physician, most of the obstacles to effective treatment can be overcome.

The most important point to remember is that most significant issues can be covered during a meeting with a physician if the information is well organized and presented in a direct, clear manner. Physicians are trained to take in and process large amounts of information in relatively short periods of time. The key to a successful meeting with a physician is for the patient to have a well-organized, carefully prepared outline that covers all the important items he or she wishes to discuss.

As a patient advocate, the first step you can take to help patients have more productive and satisfying meetings with their physicians is to aid them as they prepare for their meetings. There are two forms you and those you will be assisting can use to prepare for visits to the doctor: a patient information sheet and a patient check sheet.

PATIENT INFORMATION SHEET

The patient information sheet (see Appendix C) can be completed before the appointment and taken to the meeting with the doctor. This sheet can help you organize the information the physician needs and establish a prioritized problem list. You can explain the value of this form to the patient and assist him or her in filling it out. At the appointment, it can be handed to the doctor or you or the patient can use it to guide the discussion with the doctor. As you work with this form, be sure to explore all the issues the patient wishes to discuss and then set your priorities. Several sections of this form deserve special comment and are discussed next.

Advance Directives

If you discover that the patient does not know about advance directives or has not yet completed the appropriate forms, briefly describe the reasons he or she should consider using them and volunteer to provide additional information about them. General information about advance directives is provided in chapter 10. More detailed information and sample forms can be obtained at your local hospital. If you learn that the patient has completed advance directive forms, ask if he or she has discussed them with family members. Although the properly completed and witnessed forms are important, it is best if family members are aware of the patient's wishes. Also encourage the patient to discuss the directives with his or her doctor. The patient needs to be certain that he or she has considered all the medical situations that may be encountered, and that his or her physician understands and will honor the directives.

Medications

Patients sometimes fail to inform their physician of all the medications they are taking, especially nonprescription drugs. Be sure to obtain a complete list; the doctor needs to have this information.

Incontinence

The subject of incontinence can be difficult to discuss, but it should be addressed. Patients often neglect to mention this problem to their physician, perhaps because they find it an embarrassing subject or believe there is little that can be done to treat it. Usually the easiest way to handle this topic is to first inform the patient that incontinence is a relatively common problem for older adults, but that frequently it is overlooked during appointments. Then you can ask the patient if he or she has ever experienced this problem.

PATIENT CHECK SHEET

The patient check sheet (see Appendix D) is used as a supplement to the patient information sheet. This form can guide you as you talk with the patient and help him or her prepare for an appointment. In most cases, this form does not need to be taken to each appointment with the doctor; the information you gather as you complete this form can be concisely summarized and transferred to the patient information sheet. However, as you fill out the patient check sheet, if you discover that there have been several significant changes in the patient's life since his or her last doctor's visit, it may be best to take both the patient information sheet and the patient check sheet to the next appointment.

Frequently the information requested in the last three sections of the patient check sheet (changes in relationships or financial status, living situation, and activities of daily living) is not mentioned during visits with the doctor, yet it can be very important information. If any of this information strikes you as potentially having an effect on the patient's health, safety, or ability to obtain medical care, be sure to encourage the patient to bring it to the doctor's attention.

THE PATIENT ADVOCATE'S ROLE
IN THE MEETING WITH THE PHYSICIAN

When you and the patient have completed the patient check sheet and the patient information sheet, you need to discuss what your role will be at the doctor's office or hospital. Some patients will want you to accompany them into their meeting with the doctor to assist them in explaining their concerns and help them record the doctor's explanations and recommendations. In such situations, it is best for the patient to send the doctor a letter in advance to explain that a patient advocate will also be present for the appointment and what he or she will be doing. Exhibit 2 presents a sample letter. When you and the patient meet with the doctor, explain again who you are and why you are there. Also mention that you will excuse yourself during the physical examination, but that you would like to be brought back into the meeting so that you can hear the doctor's recommendations.

A form entitled "Summary Form for Physician Visit" (see Appendix E) can be used for recording the doctor's explanations and recommendations. Because the goal of recording the doctor's recommendations is to facilitate the accurate and complete exchange of information, it is important that you ask the physician to review and confirm what you have written down. Have the doctor initial the form on the line provided at the bottom.

Another way you can assist the patient is to encourage him or her to be assertive in expressing concerns to the doctor. Many patients find it difficult to be assertive with their physicians. Some feel that it is disrespectful to question the doctor's opinions and recommendations or to offer information that is not specifically requested. Instead, these patients adopt a passive role, allowing their doctor to ask all the questions and set the direction for discussion. They see their doctor as the source of all knowledge and expertise. Other patients are seriously skeptical of their doctor's advice, but

---

Exhibit 2. Sample Letter to Physician

Dear Dr. _____: Date: _____

As you know, my health is very important to me, and I wish to receive the very best care from you and the other health professionals I see. I am quite satisfied with the treatment and care you provide, but I realize that I also have an important role in obtaining good medical care and maintaining my health. It is my responsibility to give you all the information you need about any symptoms and illnesses, and it is also my responsibility to understand and follow the recommendations that you give me.

In an effort to better fulfill my responsibilities as a patient, I have asked a volunteer patient advocate, _____, to accompany me to my next appointment. She or he has been trained by physicians and other health care professionals at _____ (name of hospital) to provide the type of assistance a concerned relative provides for a loved one with medical problems. She or he will help me prepare a list of symptoms and concerns I can share with you at the beginning of our appointment, and she or he will help me record what you recommend. She or he has also offered to assist me in complying with your advice and treatments.

I hope you will not feel uncomfortable with this. I simply feel that I need an extra pair of eyes and ears to help me be a better patient.

Thank you for your assistance and understanding.

Sincerely,

they do not share their feelings directly with the doctor. They keep their opinions to themselves during their appointment, but once they leave, they disregard the doctor's recommendations.

Although it may seem obvious that patients need to express themselves while meeting with their physicians, we all need to recognize that it is not easy for some people to be assertive, especially with authority figures who seem to be so knowledgeable. It is important for patients to realize that they also possess valuable expertise when the subject is their health. They need to remember that they have important information that needs to be communicated to their physician, and that good, comprehensive care can be provided only when they share this information. Gentle reminders from you can help patients become more assertive.

17

After Meeting
with the Physician

The doctor's visit is an absolutely essential part of good medical care. However, for most chronic conditions, what takes place at home is just as important as what takes place in the doctor's office or hospital. In fact, most of the actual care takes place at home. For example, the medications prescribed by the doctor will be of little benefit if they are not taken correctly. Patient advocates can assist by helping patients organize their medications and providing reminders.

ASSISTING WITH MEDICATION MANAGEMENT

Noncompliance with taking prescribed medications is one of the most difficult problems physicians encounter. As many as half of patients fail to take their medications as prescribed. The problem may be even greater for many older adults, who are likely to have multiple chronic diseases and thus multiple medications.

There are many reasons why people fail to take medications as prescribed by their physician. Often patients do not understand why their doctor has prescribed a certain medication, or they do not know the purpose or benefits of the medication. They also may not know the risks of not taking the medication. In addition, often patients who experience unpleasant side effects stop taking their medication without informing their physician.

As a patient advocate, you can play a valuable role in helping patients benefit from the medications that have been prescribed. In fact, physicians consider this one of the most important roles for patient advocates. Here are several suggestions you can follow to improve patient compliance with taking medications:

- Ask the patient, Do you understand why your physician has prescribed the medication? The patient should know what the medication is for, how to take it, and what to expect. If the patient does not understand why the medication was prescribed, encourage him or her to check with the physician.
- Write down the information and instructions provided by the patient's physician. Take notes while you are in the doctor's office. Space is provided on the "Summary Form for Physician Visit" (see Appendix E).
- Encourage the patient to ask his or her primary care physician to review all the patient's medications. Suggest that the patient take all his or her medications, or at least a list of the medications, to the doctor's appointment. Include over-the-counter (nonprescription) drugs.
- Advise the patient to report any unexpected or unpleasant side effects to the doctor.
- Suggest that the patient use one pharmacist or pharmacy for all his or her medications and encourage the patient to accept medication counseling when it is offered by the pharmacist.
- Advise the patient to ask his or her pharmacist to contact the doctor when a medication is too expensive. A less expensive alternative may be available.
- Encourage the patient to use medication organizers or pillboxes.
- Help the patient keep a record of his or her medications. The record should include information about the medication, what it is for, its color and shape, the time it is to be taken, any concerns or problems related to it, and how regularly the patient takes it as prescribed. Appendix F provides a sample medication record.

Most important, encourage the patient to communicate openly with his or her physician about medications. The patient should not hesitate to ask questions or report difficulties with the medication.

Exhibit 3. Home Safety Checklist

Stairways, Hallways, and Pathways
_____ These areas have good lighting and are free from clutter.
_____ The carpet is firmly attached.
_____ Throw rugs have been removed or are firmly attached to the floor.
_____ Floors have not been waxed.
_____ Lighting is adequate at night, especially along the pathway to the bathroom.
_____ Tightly fastened handrails run the whole length and along both sides of all stairs, and light switches are at the top and bottom of all stairs.

Living Areas
_____ Cords and wires have been removed from the floor or have been placed away from walking paths.
_____ Low furniture or objects on the floor have been removed or arranged so that they are not in the way.
_____ Chairs and couches that are too low to sit in have been removed.
_____ Telephones can be easily reached.

Bathrooms
_____ Grab bars have been installed in and out of the tubs and showers and near toilets.
_____ Throw rugs have nonskid backing.
_____ Raised toilet seats have been installed.
_____ Nightlights are present.

Bedrooms
_____ Nightlights or light switches are within reach of the bed.
_____ A telephone is near the bed and within easy reach.

Outdoors
_____ Handrails have been installed on the steps and stairs.
_____ Cracked sidewalks have been repaired.
_____ Shrubbery along the pathway to the house has been trimmed.
_____ Adequate lighting has been installed by doorways and along walkways leading to the doors.

HOME SAFETY: PREVENTING ACCIDENTS AND FALLS

Patient advocates can provide valuable assistance to patients by helping them reduce their risk of falls and accidents at home by using the checklist in Exhibit 3 to evaluate their home.

THE LAITY AT WORK IN THE CONGREGATION AND COMMUNITY

18

Building the Program
within the Congregation

No aspect of our work has been more rewarding or uplifting than our interactions with outstanding congregational volunteers. At the outset we hoped to identify members of congregations who would be capable of serving as vital links between hospitals and religious institutions, but we had no idea just how talented and effective they would prove to be. We soon discovered that our health ministry program attracted individuals who brought not only valuable personal experiences and skills to their work but also tremendous energy. Their passion for this work was especially noteworthy and contagious. They energized one another, and they energized the health care professionals who were assisting with the program. Many of the professionals who provided the training for the volunteers and who served as guest speakers at congregational programs commented on how gratifying it was to work side by side with congregational lay leaders so strongly committed to enhancing community health. Doctors, nurses, pharmacists, psychologists, and other professionals reported they felt that their ability to help and heal had been greatly magnified through the efforts of the lay health educators and patient advocates.

How did we find these remarkable volunteers? And what experiences and attributes did they bring to their work? The approach we took in recruiting volunteers was to start by asking clergy to identify "natural leaders" within their congregations who might be interested in coordinating health education programs or working on a one-to-one basis as patient advocates. We explained to clergy what we wished to accomplish and what we could offer the volunteers in the way of training and resources. We felt that clergy were in a good position to evaluate both the strengths of potential leaders and the needs of their congregations. Some clergy initially were uncertain that they could find volunteers within their congregations who would be interested in this type of program and who would be effective coordinators for health programs. Nonetheless, they generally found that once they shared information about the program with key laypersons and word of the program spread throughout the congregation, one or more members would express interest and offer to attend the training programs. It became clear that this type of program has a strong attraction for certain individuals. In fact, often people in other congregations and community organizations heard about these programs and asked to participate.

Our approach to recruiting volunteers to participate in health ministries worked well. Each time we met with a new group of volunteers, we found a rich mixture of talented and motivated individuals representing a wide range of personal and vocational experiences. We found nurses, nursing assistants, teachers, social workers, small business owners, real estate agents, salespersons, and many others who were interested in the program. Some were retired whereas others were still employed. Some worked, or had worked, in private, for-profit enterprises, whereas others came out of the public or nonprofit sector. Most were active in other religious or altruistic endeavors, serving as deacons, elders, or church schoolteachers or volunteering in programs such as Habitat for Humanity. However, for some volunteers, their involvement with a health ministry program represented their first major leadership role within their congregation.

In spite of the considerable diversity within the groups, we found several common attributes among the volunteers. Perhaps most notable was their sense of altruism. It was clear that these individuals had a strong concern for the well-being of people and that they were interested in finding new ways they could help others. Many reported that they were attracted to the training program because they felt that it would better equip them to be of help and service to their congregation and community.

The volunteers also showed a deep appreciation for the value of education and recognized the critical role education can play in helping people maintain their health and independence. They were eager to learn about important health matters from professionals and just as eager to share this knowledge with members of their congregation and others in the community.

Another prominent characteristic was that the volunteers all seemed to enjoy reaching out to and interacting directly with people who shared their interest in health or who needed assistance. Before and after most training sessions, they talked with one another and exchanged ideas and information about how they could help individuals in need. Many spoke openly about their own personal experiences and how these experiences had motivated them to reach out and offer support and assistance. This motivation to reach out to people was so strong among the volunteers attending one of the training programs that they adopted the name Project REACH (Reaching out through Education to Advance Community Health) as their group name and used outstretched hands as the logo on posters and flyers announcing their congregational programs.

It is easy to see why we found it so gratifying to work with volunteers drawn from various religious congregations. These were individuals who were strongly motivated to help others, saw the value of education, and genuinely enjoyed reaching out to and having direct contact with people who needed assistance and support.

One of the outstanding volunteers we have come to know well is Barbara Pearson, a lay health educator associated with the program sponsored by Florida Hospital. Barbara, with the strong support of her pastor and other members of her church, has created an exemplary congregational and community health education program, now in its fourth year. After learning about her many successes and hearing her speak to clergy about her work, we asked Barbara to share her experiences with a larger audience by writing a chapter for this book. We feel that her words express better than ours the potential and value of a congregational health ministry program.

It is important to note that Barbara did not bring any formal training or experience in health care to her work as a lay health educator. But Barbara liked the idea of establishing a health ministry within her church, and she was willing to take the lead in developing such a program. It is evident that she brought many valuable experiences and personal qualities to her work.

Among Barbara's many valuable attributes is a strong desire to help others and a belief that if she commits herself to a worthwhile project, and does her best to make it a high-quality project, she can make a difference in the lives of others. To be certain that a program achieves a high level of quality, Barbara is willing to invest time in both the planning and implementation of the program.

Another important quality that contributes to Barbara's success is her willingness to acknowledge and draw on some of the difficult life experiences she has had. She has been able to use these experiences to deepen her understanding of health issues and connect with others who are experiencing painful or challenging health-related problems. Barbara knows what it is like for a family to face serious health problems and to need the help and support of both the medical and religious communities.

Finally, any discussion of the special qualities Barbara brings to her work in her congregation's health ministry would be incomplete without mention of her religious faith and love for her church. As you can see when you read her words, these clearly play an important part in her work.

Barbara's experiences and qualities, combined with the training and resources offered by Florida Hospital and the strong support of her pastor, have resulted in a program that continues to enhance the health of many in her congregation and that has added a new dimension to the life of a church already committed to ministering actively to the needs of its members and the greater community.

19

The Challenges and Rewards
of a Lay Health Educator Program

Barbara Pearson

My involvement in the Lay Health Educators Program has been an experience of personal growth and awareness. My association with a concept developed by faculty from two fine institutions of higher education, Stetson University and the Johns Hopkins University, is an honor. Because my husband and I have one daughter who graduated from Stetson University and another daughter who graduated from Johns Hopkins University, I am doubly proud to participate in this creative and caring ministry. The standard of excellence that both Stetson and Johns Hopkins are known for further validates the Lay Health Educators Program.

I view my participation in this program as a ministry, and it has reinforced my belief that members of a religious congregation can be effective ministers. For some time I have believed in the strength of the laity being involved in the work of the church, and I have come to see the involvement of lay workers in the area of community health as particularly valuable. I am fortunate to be a member of College Park Baptist Church, a church that allows its members to find and use their spiritual gifts. Our church is privileged to have as members Dr. and Mrs. Findley Edge. Dr. Edge taught at Southern Seminary in Louisville, Kentucky, for more than forty years and distinguished himself as a professor and an author of several books. Those familiar with him know of his belief that each congregational member is called to be a minister and of his passion for the laity at work in the church and the world. Referring to the professional minister, he states:

> Ministers are pulled asunder by the overwhelming and sometimes conflicting demands made upon them. They are to preach. They are to evangelize. They are to engage in social action. They are to administer. They are to visit. They are to counsel. For them to attempt to do all these alone is impossible from the human perspective and erroneous from the biblical perspective. The pastor's ministry is to equip the saints for the work of the ministry. (Edge 1994, 70)

Dr. Edge goes on to describe the work that the laity, or "saints," should do. He believes that the church needs to be attuned to the social issues that confront our communities. Among these are the health needs of the community. He states, "The Christian must have a deep concern for the health conditions in the community. This concern may begin in one's own community, but it must reach out to people living in all the world" (Edge 1994, 85). I share this view, and I believe that the laity, working closely with pastors and health care professionals, can play a critical and an influential part in addressing the health needs of our communities.

The medical community is deeply concerned that the public receives correct and understandable information on medical matters. My husband is a physician, and I know of his acute concern for the accurate dispensing of medical facts. A high level of trust is developed when the integrity of the church is combined with that of medical professionals who are willing to participate and share time and expertise in their field. A vast amount of information is not easily accessible or understood by laypersons. The Lay Health Educators Program strives to provide laypersons with easy-to-understand, pertinent, and correct information in a timely manner. How much better to learn this information from the medical professional than television news programs or magazine articles that, at best, do not present a clear picture of the issues. The layperson, therefore, can become an asset to the medical community as well as the church in helping create medical awareness and insight.

The church and the medical community are natural partners in the disbursement of medical information. Jesus was greatly concerned for both the spiritual and physical health of the lives he touched. A. T. Robertson (1950) lists in *A Harmony of the Gospels* thirty-five miracles performed by Jesus; twenty-five are healing miracles. The church, following the example of Jesus, can be an extension of the medical community as a place of compassion and caring, concerned with the whole person. I believe the ministry of the Lay Health Educators Program is completely consistent with the teachings of Jesus.

A positive outcome I have observed in this program is an increased rapport between the medical community and the layperson. Some laypersons may not have had an opportunity to discuss health matters with professionals outside of an examining room or hospital setting. To know that the physician or another health care professional has given time, shared in a question-and-answer period, and been willing to stay beyond the scheduled session can only serve to improve the public's trust and confidence in the medical community.

With the presentation of good medical knowledge, church members can learn the importance of individual responsibility in their health matters. They can learn that steps can be taken to help prevent the onset of certain health problems and that it is important to comply properly with recommended treatment in order to lessen the impact of chronic conditions.

INGREDIENTS FOR SUCCESS

There are some necessary ingredients for having a successful lay health educators program. First, it is imperative to have a supportive pastor, one who allows laypersons to offer suggestions for a church program and then provides the support they need to implement the program. Dr. Charles Horton, pastor of College Park Baptist Church, has been an enthusiastic supporter of my work. Even before we had our first series in 1996, he allowed time in the Sunday worship hour for presentations on the importance of being an organ donor and on living wills. As a "kick-off" to our first health series, he preached a sermon, "The Theology of Health," in which he challenged the congregation to make a personal commitment to a biblical view of health and to see the body as a precious gift of God. For the last four years, Dr. Horton has given time each Wednesday night in January for this special medical focus, and he has graciously allowed announcements to be made in the Sunday worship hour. He believes in the program and has seen the positive response of our congregation.

Second, it is important to have a lay health educator who truly cares for the members of the church. I went to the first class held at Florida Hospital/Orlando not really understanding what was involved. After the first session, I was highly stimulated by the classes and looked forward to each one. There I met others who cared deeply about the needs of their fellow members. As the weeks passed, I became more convinced that this program was something I wanted to make available to my church. I wanted the members of my church to have the same kind of information I had been privileged to receive. I greatly wanted people to make lifestyle changes to help prevent certain diseases. I wanted them to be aware of physical symptoms that might alert them to seek medical attention and lead to early detection. I wanted them to know the hope of treatments and resources available for a better quality of life. And I wanted them to realize the need to be responsible, take control of their health, and comprehend the necessity of complying with medical recommendations.

Third, members of the congregation who serve as lay health educators need to have good organizational skills and enjoy coordinating projects. In planning a series of seminars or other programs, juggling of schedules is required when requesting extremely busy professionals to give their time on a specific date. My interchange with each prospective speaker gave me an opportunity to describe and talk about the program. In spite of their busy schedules, I found that the professionals I asked to participate in our program were extremely impressed with this innovative idea for giving medical information. They felt that their time participating in the program was well spent.

Last, the continued support and interest of a sponsoring health care institution is invaluable. In our case, Dr. Dan Hale of Stetson University and staff from Florida Hospital have provided encouragement and numerous resources throughout the program. Joan Salmons, the senior executive officer for clinical services at Florida Hospital and the driving force behind the hospital's sponsorship of the program, came to College Park Baptist Church on two occasions to make a special announcement about our medical series. She was accompanied by Shelly Siebenlist, the nurse and hospital administrator who had coordinated the initial training program. The presence of these two hospital representatives gave further credibility and importance to what we were trying to do. Follow-up meetings and dinners given for those who took the classes at Florida Hospital have continued to keep interest alive and indicate that those individuals believe in us and are appreciative of our efforts.

THE ONGOING SUCCESS OF THE PROGRAM

The response of College Park Baptist Church has been both positive and encouraging. We have now completed our fourth year of involvement in this program. There has never been a time that someone has not said to me, "Thank you so much for bringing someone to discuss this topic. I have this problem or a member of my family suffers from this disease, and tonight I learned so much."

We have appreciated the good attendance. We had no idea how many to expect because we had never had such an event. The first year an average of 90 persons attended each of the five sessions, with a total attendance for the series of more than 450 persons. Attendance has remained good for each series. We gave a survey following the first group of programs and were pleased to have 66 persons complete it. Included in the survey was the question, "Do you hope to make some lifestyle changes?" Fifty-nine responded "yes" to this question. The response was both significant and rewarding because it indicated that we had made a difference in our church members' lives.

In the survey, we allowed space for comments. The comments were highly complimentary. The most significant statement came from a 32-year-old mother of two. She said, "I am so proud of our church for providing this 'inreach' program to our members. I feel you ministered to a need in my life, and that is to better understand these health issues. I recently lost both of my parents to heart disease that was undetected in both. I greatly appreciated the opportunity to hear these speakers. It not only was informative, but will help our family plan for a healthy future."

That first survey listed additional topics for consideration as future programs and provided an area for people to select those of most interest.

Those topics were then used for the next two series. After the third year of health education programs, we again gave a survey to determine the interest of continuing this type of education. We found a decided interest in more medical seminars. It seems to me that people are vitally interested in obtaining medical knowledge, especially when it is sponsored by their church.

Although most of our participants were senior adults, we did encourage adults of all ages to attend, and we always had younger adults present. Prevention measures need to begin early, so I believe these programs should be available to all age groups. In fact, in our fourth year we included programs aimed at teenagers and their parents.

OUR PROGRAM'S CURRICULUM

The following is a list of topics covered in the four years of our lay health education program:

- Orthopedics
- Heart disease
- Malignant diseases
- Diet/nutrition
- When to seek the help of a psychiatrist
- Depression
- Managed care
- Diabetes
- Medication management
- Alcoholism as a disease
- Recovery for the alcoholic and the family
- Alzheimer disease
- Advance directives
- Dermatology
- Teenage stress and depression
- Substance abuse (one program for youth alone and another for youth and parents)
- Alcoholism (talk given to youth by a young adult recovering alcoholic)

Alcoholism may seem like a difficult or questionable subject to cover in a church-sponsored program on health. Many people are reluctant to consider alcoholism as a medical condition requiring professional treatment, even though it has long been recognized as a disease within the medical community. Others may believe it is a problem that is relatively uncommon among members of their congregation. The fact is, alcoholism is a serious and pervasive problem that affects, either directly or indirectly, large numbers of church-going people. It is an illness that affects our teenagers, the adult population, and, at increasingly alarming rates, our elderly. Alcoholism is a chronic and progressive illness that can lead to the destruction of families, financial ruin, and even death unless detected and treated.

Alcoholism is a family disease, because it deeply affects every member. A conservative estimate is that at least ten persons are affected by each alcoholic. One can see the overwhelming magnitude of the devastating effect not only on the alcoholic but on the family and friends as well.

Because there is hope for the individuals and families who recognize the serious nature of alcoholism and who seek appropriate treatment, we felt it was a topic we should cover in our health education series. We had two speakers—one from Alcoholics Anonymous (AA) and one from Al-Anon, the support group for family and friends of alcoholics. In our most recent series, we had a young adult recovering alcoholic speak about his experiences. I like what Frederick Buechner (1991) says about AA and Al-Anon. He believes that churches can learn much from these groups. He says that "what goes on in them is far closer to what Christ meant his church to be, and what it originally was, than much of what goes on in most churches I know" (93). He notes that "the one thing they [group members] have in common can be easily stated. It is just that they all believe that they cannot live fully human lives without each other and without what they call their Higher Power" (90–91). I am a passionate believer in these simple, but profound and beautiful groups. And I am a grateful member of Al-Anon.

A PROGRAM OF ADVOCACY AND SUPPORT

Another wonderful program for assisting senior adults in our churches has been developed—the Patient Advocacy Program. This program trains people to be a second set of eyes and ears for older adults who have no family members or friends to accompany them to their doctor's appointment. Recommendations and medications can be misunderstood at any age, but especially by the elderly, who are likely to have multiple health problems and be taking numerous medications. Patient advocates can provide comfort for patients and ensure that they properly understand their medical treatment.

Certainly churches care for the needs of people. How to meet those needs is a challenge, but what better place than a church to supply information for both spiritual and physical healing. Here is where lay leaders can give guidance in the same way as laity lead in other areas of church life. I think of the compassionate hands of Jesus and see laity and pastors, together, ministering the healing medicine of compassion, love, involvement, comfort, encouragement, and understanding. Henri Nouwen, in his book *The Wounded Healer*, speaks of the healing power of such a ministry: "When we become aware that we do not have to escape our pains, but that we can mobilize them into a common search for life, those very pains are transformed from expressions of despair into signs of hope" (1979, 93). We can share in our problems whether they are spiritual, physical, or emotional.

I also believe that people need to be touched by loving hands, and I wish to be available to reach out and touch them. They need to know I am there as a source of human presence in their hour of need. The woman who reached out to touch Jesus' garment believed, "If I could just touch his garment, I would be made whole." That miracle was an illustration of her great faith, but I believe that I need to develop the sensitivity that makes me open to be touched and provide others with the human touch that each of us needs, even when God is there. I believe the lay health education and the patient advocacy programs are very practical avenues for both touching lives and making oneself available to be touched.

Wouldn't it be exciting and rewarding to know that we had helped people in our congregations to implement lifestyle changes that might prevent or decrease the risk of disease, and to learn to recognize symptoms, seek treatment, and then comply with the prescribed treatment, leading to a better quality of living and maybe even preventing an early death? I am grateful for the vision of Dr. Dan Hale, Dr. John Burton, Dr. Richard Bennett, Joan Salmons, and their colleagues at Stetson University, the Johns Hopkins University, and Florida Hospital, as well as all the others who helped develop this idea. Surely God was in the plan from the beginning.

REFERENCES

Buechner, F. 1991. *Telling Secrets*. New York: HarperCollins.
Edge, F. B. 1994. *A Quest for Vitality in Religion*. Macon, Ga.: Smith & Helwys.
Nouwen, H. J. M. 1979. *The Wounded Healer*. New York: Doubleday.
Robertson, A. T. 1950. *A Harmony of the Gospels*. New York: Harper & Brothers.

APPENDIXES

Appendix A

Congregational Survey

We are interested in organizing some programs on health-related topics that are of interest to members of the congregation. You can help us plan for these programs by completing this brief survey. Please place a check by topics that you would be interested in learning more about.

_____ Adolescent health issues

_____ Alcohol abuse

_____ Anxiety disorders

_____ Arthritis

_____ Cancer

_____ Cardiopulmonary resuscitation (CPR)

_____ Dementia/Alzheimer disease

_____ Depression

_____ Diabetes

_____ Exercise and health

_____ Eye diseases/vision problems

_____ Heart disease

_____ Hypertension

_____ Living wills/advance directives

_____ Medications

_____ Men's health issues

_____ Nutrition and health

_____ Orthopedic problems

_____ Pain management

_____ Prevention of accidents and falls

_____ Respiratory disorders

_____ Sleep disorders

_____ Stress management

_____ Vaccinations (influenza and pneumonia)

_____ Women's health issues

Suggestions

_____

_____

_____

_____

_____

_____

Appendix B

Program Evaluation Form

We would greatly appreciate your taking the time to complete this brief questionnaire. By doing so, you can help us plan for future programs.

I found this program to be informative and helpful.
___ Strongly agree   ___ Agree   ___ Disagree   ___ Strongly disagree

Based on what I learned in this program, I feel better equipped to handle health matters.
___ Strongly agree   ___ Agree   ___ Disagree   ___ Strongly disagree

What could have been done to make this program better?

_____

_____

_____

_____

_____

What topic(s) would you like covered in future programs?

_____

_____

_____

_____

_____

Other suggestions or comments?

_____

_____

_____

_____

_____

Appendix C

Patient Information Sheet

Date: _____

Name: _____ Phone: _____

Surrogate (and relationship): _____

   Phone: _____

Advocate: _____

Advance directives: _____

Allergies: _____

Pharmacy: _____ Phone: _____

Current Medications

Prescribed Drugs	*Dosage and Frequency*
_____	_____
_____	_____
_____	_____
_____	_____
_____	_____
_____	_____

Over-the-Counter Drugs	*Dosage and Frequency*
_____	_____
_____	_____
_____	_____
_____	_____
_____	_____
_____	_____

Patient needs assistance with these basic and instrumental activities of daily living:

_____

_____

_____

_____

Incontinence problems: Bladder? Yes No   Bowel? Yes No   (circle answers)

Other concerns:

_____

_____

_____

_____

Prioritized Problem List

1. _____
2. _____
3. _____
4. _____
5. _____

Appendix D

Patient Check Sheet

Name: _____   Date: _____

How do you rate your health? ___ excellent ___ good ___ fair ___ poor

Have you been hospitalized in the last year? ___no ___1 time ___2 –3 times
___more than 3 times

Have you used an emergency room in the last year? ___ yes ___ no

Vaccination status (date last received):

Influenza_____

Pneumococcal _____

Tetanus _____

Symptom review (check if a problem):

_____ Visual difficulties

_____ Hearing difficulties

_____ Forgetfulness

_____ Sleeping problems

_____ Depression or loss of interest in usual activities

_____ Other types of emotional distress

_____ Urinary incontinence/leakage

_____ Fecal (bowel movement) incontinence

Have you experienced the following events in the last year? (circle answers and describe if yes)

Yes   No   Death of a spouse _____

Yes   No   Death of other close family member _____

Yes   No   Marriage or new companion _____

Yes   No   Change in financial status _____

Yes   No   Change in living situation _____

Yes   No   Loss of long-time pet(s)_____

Yes   No   Divorce or separation _____

Living situation:

_____ House   _____ Apartment   _____ Other

_____ Alone   _____ With other person(s)

List important aspects of your living situation: _____

_____

Difficulties with basic and instrumental activities of daily living:

_____ Walking or moving

_____ Using the toilet

_____ Managing medications

_____ Bathing

_____ Personal grooming

_____ Managing money

_____ Shopping

_____ Dressing

_____ Preparing meals

_____ Housekeeping

_____ Transferring (into and out of bed or chair)

_____ Using the telephone

_____ Eating

Appendix E

Summary Form for Physician Visit

Physician's assessment of overall health status:

_____ Same _____ Improved _____ Worsened

New problems identified by physician:

_____

_____

_____

_____

_____

New medications or changes in previous therapy:

_____

_____

_____

_____

_____

Other physicians who need to be seen for consultation:

Name: _____

Telephone: _____

Address: _____

Date of appointment: _____

Time of appointment: _____

Name: _____

Telephone: _____

Address: _____

Date of appointment: _____

Time of appointment: _____

Tests that need to be done before the next visit:

Name of test: _____

Location: _____

Telephone: _____

Date of appointment: _____

Time of appointment: _____

Name of test: _____

Location: _____

Telephone: _____

Date of appointment: _____

Time of appointment: _____

Other instructions: _____

_____

_____

_____

_____

Next appointment (date and time): _____

Reviewed by (physician's initials): _____

Appendix F

Medication Record

Name: _____ Date: _____ Completed by: _____

Primary physician's name: _____ Physician's telephone number: _____

Prescribed Medication	What Is It For?	Pill Size (e.g., 5 mg, 1 capsule)	Color and Shape	Time Taken (e.g., 8 A.M., 12 noon)	Concerns or Problems	Compliance (e.g., always, sometimes, never)

Suggested Readings

RELIGION AND HEALTH

Herbert Benson. *Timeless Healing: The Power and Biology of Belief.* New York: Scribner, 1996.

Harold G. Koenig. *The Healing Power of Faith: Science Explores Medicine's Last Great Frontier.* New York: Simon & Schuster, 1999.

Dale A. Mathews. *The Faith Factor: Proof of the Healing Power of Prayer.* New York: Viking Press, 1998.

HEALTH BELIEF MODEL

I. M. Rosenstock. Historical origins of the health belief model. *Health Education Monographs* 2 (1974): 328–35.

MOTIVATIONAL INTERVIEWING

William R. Miller and Stephen Rollnick. *Motivational Interviewing: Preparing People to Change Addictive Behavior.* New York: Guilford Press, 1991.

MEDICAL RESOURCES

Michael J. Klag. *Johns Hopkins Family Health Book.* New York: HarperCollins, 1999.

The Johns Hopkins Medical Letter Health after 50. Subscription Department, P.O. Box 420179, Palm Coast, Fla. 32142; tel. (904) 446-4675.

DEPRESSION AND MENTAL DISORDERS

Rosalynn Carter. *Helping Someone with Mental Illness.* New York: Times Books, 1999.

Kay Redfield Jamison. *An Unquiet Mind.* New York: Vintage Books, 1996.

Martha Manning. *Undercurrents: A Life beneath the Surface.* New York: HarperCollins, 1996.

William Styron. *Darkness Visible: A Memoir of Madness.* New York: Vintage Books, 1992.

DEMENTIA

Nancy L. Mace and Peter V. Rabins. *The 36-Hour Day: A Family Guide to Caring for Persons with Alzheimer Disease, Related Dementing Illnesses, and Memory Loss in Later Life*, 3d ed. Baltimore: Johns Hopkins University Press, 1999.

Index

Printed in the United States
82366LV00003B/178